HEARST MARINE BOOKS
GUIDE TO
FRESHWATER
FISHING BOATS

HEARST MARINE BOOKS GUIDE TO FRESHWATER FISHING BOATS

Mike Toth

Illustrations by Ron Carboni

HEARST MARINE BOOKS
New York

Library of Congress Cataloging-in-Publication Data

Hearst Marine Books guide to freshwater fishing boats / Mike Toth ; illustrations
    by Ron Carboni.
        p.   cm.
    Includes index.
    ISBN 0-688-13733-4
    1. Fishing boats—Design and construction. 2. Fishing boats—Equipment and supplies.
3. Fishing—Equipment and supplies.
    VM431.H43   1995
    623.8'231'0247991—dc20   95-13718
                                                                 CIP

Printed in the United States of America

First Edition

1 2 3 4 5 6 7 8 9 10

Produced for Hearst Books by
Michael Mouland & Associates,
Toronto

Typesetting and page layout by Tom Sankey

ACKNOWLEDGMENTS

This book would not have been possible without the kind and generous assistance of many people. Many thanks to Anthony Acerrano, Monte Burch, Frank Golad, Geri Haber, Chuck Merritt, Bruce W. Smith, and Mark Thomas. And to my father, who started me on this journey by first taking me fishing when I was four years old and who still finds the time to go out with me. And finally, thanks to my wife, Reggie, for all her cheer and support during this project, not the least of which was taking care of our two-year-old, Joey, as well as for giving birth to Caroline in the middle of Chapter 6.

CONTENTS

INTRODUCTION

The first boat I ever owned wasn't really mine. It was a twelve-foot aluminum cartopper that my father bought new (and generously called "ours") almost twenty-five years ago. I used to sit in the gleaming white skiff on cold winter mornings, the whole craft canted sideways on my parents' garage floor, dreaming about the upcoming fishing season.

The first time we used it I struggled to "help" my father take the boat off the station-wagon roof. My twelve-year-old muscles ached from half-carrying and half-dragging the boat down to the water. But I was proud of the pain; after all, it was *our* boat.

Dad and I caught a lot of fish from that little boat over the years: pickerel in New Jersey's Pine Barrens, largemouth bass in the Adirondacks, trout in the Poconos. I even took the boat with me to college one year, keeping it chained to a light-post outside my apartment.

That boat is still around, though Dad and I have gone on to bigger craft and different waters. We haven't used the old tin skiff in years, but we won't get rid of it. Sure, it holds a lot of sentimental value for both of us, but most of all we keep it for one reason: it is a very good fishing boat.

That's why I'm bothered when I hear platitudes such as "The happiest day in a fisherman's life is the day he buys a boat. The second happiest day in a fisherman's life is the day he sells it"; or "Definition of a boat: a hole in the water into which one throws money."

Obviously there are plenty of unhappy boat owners in the world. Doubt it? Pick up your local newspaper and see how many used boats are listed for sale in the classified section. Or drive to the nearest lake on a beautiful summer day and see how many boats are moored to the dock, inactive, silent.

Can you imagine making a significant financial investment in something that is supposed to give you nothing but pleasure—and ending up hating it?

Evidently you can't (or at least don't want to) because you have this book in your hands. You probably are a somewhat experienced fisherman, and you may already know a few things about boats—you might have a particular make, model, and size in mind already—but you want to learn more about fishing boats before you go out and actually buy one.

Congratulate yourself. By buying this book, you did not get ripped off, fooled, or misled. You will not regret this purchase months or years from now. This book will not sit in the side of your yard or at a slip in a marina, suffering from neglect and losing its value. You will not want to sell it to somebody else. Let's make sure that the boat you finally buy isn't a disappointment either.

Remember that no boat is absolutely perfect for all purposes. The point is to find one that best suits your specific needs. Sometime in the future you may wish to buy another boat because you want more (or possibly less) room and power, an improved design, or different capabilities.

If you do everything right the first time, *that* day will be the second happiest day of your life.

HEARST MARINE BOOKS
GUIDE TO FRESHWATER FISHING BOATS

1

THE BEST BOAT FOR YOU

Only three criteria characterize a boat: it must float, it must be large enough to hold and transport at least one person, and it must be maneuverable by that person.

If that person can drop a baited line over its side, it becomes a *fishing* boat.

A small boy straddling a log, kicking his way out to the middle of a pond to lower a bent pin baited with bread and tied to some kite string, has become the envy of his shore-bound buddies because he now is a boat fisherman. Even such a rudimentary craft can be considered a fishing boat, because it meets those four criteria. It also creates a new dimension of fishing for the small boy: He's no longer confined to fishing from the banks of the pond, where the water he can fish is limited to how far he can toss his baited line. He doesn't have to fight with his friends for the best spots. He can move from

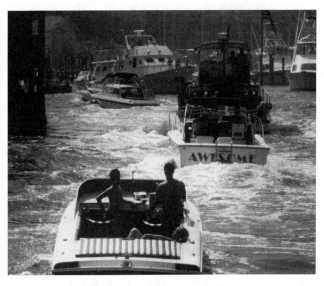

You can fish from just about any boat—and there are thousands of types on the water today—but a good freshwater fishing boat has to satisfy a number of criteria.

1

one side of the pond to the other with only a few kicks of his legs.

Mobility, maneuverability, access to better fishing: such are the basic desires that spur us to get a boat of our own—though we may want a few more features and comforts than a floating log provides.

HOW BIG?

The size parameters of boats used for fishing in freshwater are fairly wide. The shortest typical length is twelve feet, which is the average size of skiffs and johnboats that can be carried on the roof rack of a car or in the bed of a pickup truck. (Some johnboats run a foot or two smaller, and some truly "portable" boats are no more than eight feet long.) Fourteen- to sixteen-foot craft are quite common, and they provide more room and stability than do the cartoppers.

The largest typical freshwater fishing boat— and by their very size they must be restricted to use in large waters—runs about 26 feet in length and 8½ feet in width. One reason for this cutoff point concerns legality: a special permit is necessary to tow objects much wider than this on public roads. Additionally, 26-foot boats and others in that category are light enough to be towed by most large sedans, heavier pickup trucks, and sport/utility vehicles. Larger craft are used on many freshwater lakes, especially on the Great Lakes, but few of them are recreational fishing boats.

In between these two sizes lie the majority of boats in use by anglers today. The size you want depends on your personal tastes, your available finances, and your storage capacity. Just as important a factor in this decision, however, is the boat's design, which should be dictated by both the species of fish you want to catch and the type of water you'll be fishing in.

THE HULL

The configuration of the hull—the "bottom" of a boat, which contacts the water—defines a boat's applications.

The most basic hull design is the **flat bottom**. This shape hull allows easy maneuvering and is very stable in calm waters because it displaces a relatively large amount of water. Johnboats typically have flat-bottom hulls.

The **round-bottom** hull resembles a flat bottom with rounded angles (called chines) where the bottom and sides meet. Round bottoms offer even more ease of maneuverability than do flat bottoms.

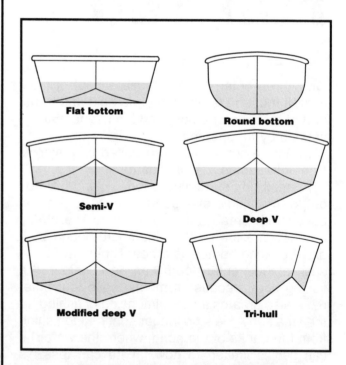

These six hull shapes are the most common on freshwater fishing boats. All offer different handling characteristics, advantages, and disadvantages.

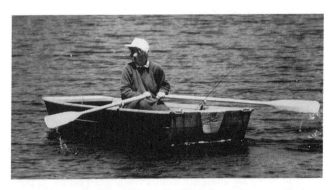

Flat-bottomed hulls are easy to maneuver on calm, protected waters. This little craft is perfect for one angler on ponds or small lakes that don't allow outboard motors.

Two distinct disadvantages with flat- and round-bottomed hulls: they give a rough ride in even a mild chop, and they don't come up "on plane," or partially lift from the water to effect greater speed, very easily. But they're extremely well suited to calm lakes and ponds, as well as small waters where speed is not a factor. This is why many cartopping anglers own johnboats.

The remainder of hull types are called planing hulls, obviously because they are designed to come up on plane.

The *semi-V* hull resembles a flat bottom except for the shallow V shape in its forward portion. This shape allows for a bit more stability than does the flat bottom, and it attains plane easier.

The *deep-V* hull, as its name implies, is sharply angled from bow to stern. The deep V is the best hull design for use in rough water, because it "slices" through waves and swells and planes quickly. Because of the sharp angle, however, it does have more draft (it sits deeper in the water) and therefore is not suitable for fishermen who frequent the shallows. It also tends to rock at rest when hit broadside by waves.

The *modified-deep-V* hull is a shallower-angle version of the deep V. A relatively recent development, the modified deep V is an excellent compromise hull choice for an all-around fishing

boat. It comes up on plane relatively easily, and doesn't need a lot of horsepower to do so. It offers a fairly smooth ride in rough water, doesn't rock as easily as a deep V, and can enter shallower water.

The *tri-hull* (also called a *cathedral hull*) consists of three parallel V-shaped hulls. Made famous by the Boston Whaler company (though it is certainly not the only boat manufacturer to utilize this hull shape), the tri-hull offers superb stability as well as shallow draft. Some boaters complain of a jarring ride in unsettled water with a tri-hull, but because of its "go-anywhere" capability it is a popular hull choice among many experienced fishermen.

Each boat manufacturer nowadays seems to have its own special hull design. Often these are takeoffs on or adaptations of one of the hull shapes mentioned above. A cursory examination of the hull will reveal its basic form.

Sometimes certain features are added to the hull's design to make the boat more appropriate for use on a certain type of water. One popular feature on a hull, for example, is a "reversed chine," in which the angle formed where the bottom and sides meet is concave rather than convex. Such a feature is said to provide a drier ride than normal because spray is directed away from the inside of

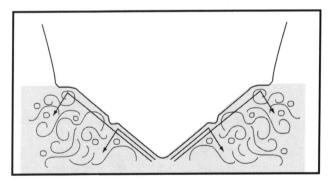

Hulls with reversed chines, such as this representation of a hull on a Grady-White boat, are supposed to direct surface spray downward to give occupants a drier ride.

the boat when under power. This is worthwhile if you expect to use the boat under predominantly rough conditions, but not necessary if you're planning to fish small, protected waters.

Remember, there are hundreds of boat manufacturers, but a boat dealer typically will stock fewer than a dozen makes of craft—sometimes just one or two. So, the hull shapes you see at one dealer may not be representative of the entire hull family. The dealer should be able to provide an adequate explanation of the hull designs on the boats carried. Ask about the specific advantages and disadvantages of each hull type, and why. As boat dealers will usually stock those types of boats that are desirable for use in nearby waters, the hulls on the boats (as well as the boats themselves) should reflect that consideration.

ALUMINUM OR FIBERGLASS?

The first boat ever made was formed of wood, and the old wooden rowboat isn't an extinct species. But wood has been supplanted by new materials that are practically maintenance-free in freshwater and are much easier to work with on a large-scale production operation.

Aluminum and fiberglass are the two predominant materials used for boat construction today. Each has its pros and cons.

Fiberglass, which in the boat industry is a general term for layers of various types of resin laid onto a wood or plastic (or wood/plastic combination) frame, is a strong material and can stand up to pounding waves quite well. It's also heavy, providing stability in certain situations, such as when carrying heavy or unbalanced loads. Its form allows for rounded angles and a generally streamlined appearance. And fiberglass is an easy material to work with once a manufacturer is set up for the process.

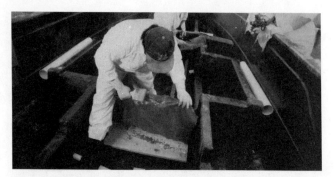

Hulls of fiberglass boats are made on molds and consist of layers of fiberglass cloth laid in with polyester resins.

The weight of fiberglass is its largest detraction, however. A fiberglass cartop boat can be quite unwieldy to load and unload (at least when compared with aluminum cartoppers). And such weight requires an accordingly larger motor to power it on the water. Buying a high-horsepower outboard may not seem like a significant financial sacrifice for owning a fiberglass boat (although many boat owners like the idea of speed anyway, or at least the idea of having power in reserve). But if you're planning to tow the boat, your vehicle may not be large enough or powerful enough to handle all that weight.

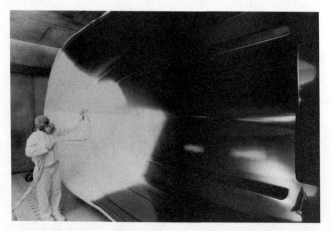

A covering of color gel-coat and clear gel-coat is applied to a fiberglass hull.

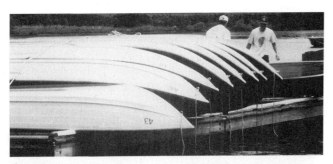

Because of their light weight, aluminum boats are easy to carry and store. The fact that many boat liveries use aluminum craft for their rentals is testimony to the substance's durability as well.

Aluminum boats, which consist of narrow-gauge sheets of the metal welded together at the seams, have become legion during the last two decades. Its light weight, rigidity, and low cost make aluminum ideal for the small- to medium-size range of freshwater fishing boats. It also is the substance that has sparked the evolution of the cartop boat. A fisherman and a friend can toss a twelve-footer on top of the family sedan, drive to the nearest lake and hand-carry it down to the shoreline—no launch ramp necessary.

But for all its attributes, aluminum isn't perfect. Its light weight makes it prone to pounding when

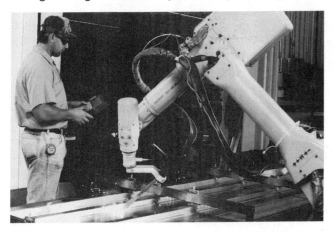

Robotic welding machines are used in the construction of Crestliner aluminum boats.

motoring through a chop, making for an uncomfortable ride. Aluminum is noisy as well. Pleasure boaters may not care about the noise factor, but watch a fisherman's reaction when a loaded tackle box clunks down onto the deck of an aluminum boat! It's not the actual noise but the vibrations that will send fish scurrying away. (Carpeting or planking will help deaden such sound waves.) Still, the noise factor of an aluminum boat is a small price to pay for such mobility.

Most aluminum fishing boats are less than eighteen feet in length. A few manufacturers have models larger than this, and their owners are quite satisfied.

KEVLAR

The material that Du Pont created has been getting most attention in its use for construction of bullet-proof vests. But the incredible strength of Kevlar, in comparison with its weight, makes it an ideal substance for a boat.

A boat made of Kevlar is only a bit heavier than the same size boat made of aluminum. On a weight-for-weight basis it is stronger than both aluminum and fiberglass, resisting impact and bending to a much higher degree. The light weight also means that less money can be spent on both boat motor and tow vehicle. But a Kevlar boat costs more than a fiberglass boat—and a lot more than an aluminum boat.

Kevlar's advantages are worthy but, considering the price factor, not important enough to the majority of the boating public for manufacturers to make all boats out of Kevlar. The research on Kevlar and other polymers continues, so at some point in the future we may see the invention of the "perfect" boat material—superstrong, superlight, supercheap. But for now, fiberglass and aluminum perform just fine for most of us.

FACTORY FEATURES: ROOM TO FISH, ROOM FOR FISH

Here's where we encounter the real difference between fishing boats and all other boats: the attributes of a particular craft that make it suitable for fishing.

Probably the most important feature of a fishing boat is its interior layout. Anglers need more than just a place to sit: we need room to stand when casting or fighting a fish or dropping an anchor; room for other fishermen; room for rods, tackle boxes, ice chests, bait, electronics, food, clothing, and—we hope, anyway—fish.

But this is not to say that fishermen need big boats. Thousands of fishermen get by quite nicely with twelve-foot utility craft. The importance lies in the design of the boat, specifically in its open-space roominess and storage capacity.

A fishing boat should be roomy for both comfort and necessity. Fishermen often spend many hours aboard their craft—all day, sometimes—so having space to shift your position, stretch your legs, and reach for gear becomes important. Sitting in one tight position for a couple of hours is enough to discourage further outings.

Johnboats, cartoppers, and the like in the twelve- to fourteen-foot range are open in design. The seating arrangement in these small boats usually consists of benches running from gunwale to gunwale with a four- or five-person capacity, but such a crowd leaves little room for either comfort or equipment. In a twelve-foot boat, for example, two or three anglers and their gear is about the maximum. These open boats usually have little true *dedicated* storage space such as holds and hatches, but the unfilled seats and deck provide plenty of room for personal movement as well as places to put gear.

Open boats in the fourteen- to seventeen-foot category usually have some type of built-in storage containers. These typically are nothing more than a hollow seat with a lidded top, but they are more than adequate for their purpose. These under-seat storage spaces are best used to keep ancillary equipment—life preservers, fire extinguisher, rope—that is necessary on any excursion but not integral to a fishing trip. You want your fishing gear immediately acessible, not stored where you must stand up and lift a lid every time you want to change a lure.

Console or cockpit boats, which usually start in the sixteen-foot range, come with dedicated storage space as well. Many of them have a *locker*, or a hollow section located somewhere in the deck, accessible via a lid. Again, such storage areas are suited to equipment that won't be constantly handled when fishing. A hold in the bow area, for example, is perfect for stowing an anchor with chain and rope attached: it's out of the way, but readily available and exactly where you need it.

Manufacturers have created ingenious storage spaces in other parts of boats, such as an ice cooler inside a gunwale and a tackle drawer system in the rear of a center-console seat. These storage spaces come in quite handy to fishermen, as tackle and gear should always be accessible and not in inconvenient places.

Another popular option on a console boat is a *livewell* or *baitwell*. Though definitions vary from manufacturer to manufacturer, a livewell is a place to keep fish that you've caught, and a baitwell is a place to keep live bait. Sometimes one well will serve dual purposes, though not simultaneously. These wells consist of a hollowed-out section of a gunwale, transom, or seat base capable of holding water—basically a conveniently integrated minnow bucket or fish box. The advantage of these built-in wells is that you don't have to change the water manually, as most baitwells/livewells offer

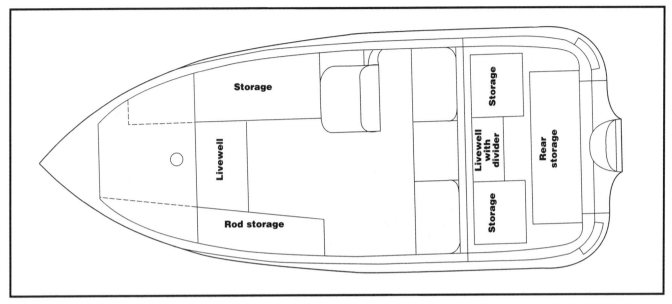

Some boats come with features designed specifically for anglers. This layout of a Ranger bass boat, for example, offers integrated storage space for fishing rods as well as dual livewells.

an automatic freshwater inflow, whether self-filling or pumped electronically. Many offer an electronic aeration system to keep bait and/or fish literally alive and kicking.

Rod holders are another convenient feature found on larger boats. There are two types: holders located on the gunwales, which hold rods upright for trolling or baitfishing; and rod holders that keep rods safely stowed out of the way when not in use.

The gunwale holders can serve both active (fishing) and passive (storage) purposes. They are nothing more than a cuplike device built into the gunwale in which the rod butt is inserted. A crosspiece located some distance down from the mouth of the holder keeps the fishing reel from banging or scraping against the gunwale itself.

Rod storage devices consist of horizontal racks located under the gunwale, which keep

them safely out of the way of arms, feet, and other rods. These racks are excellent for storing rods when trailering or for keeping extra rods on board.

Another rod storage device, commonly known as a *rocket launcher* because rods sit upright and close together in it, is located on the console, tower, or stern of larger boats. This keeps rods stored out of the way of active fishermen on board but convenient enough that they can be grabbed quickly when they are needed.

Generally, the larger the boat, the more standard fishing features are built into it. The price tag of the boat increases accordingly. Fortunately, many of these handy items can be added to your boat separately. (A large ice chest, for example, doesn't have to be used only for keeping cold and wet things cold and wet. It also keeps dry things dry—tackle, clothing, electronic equipment—just

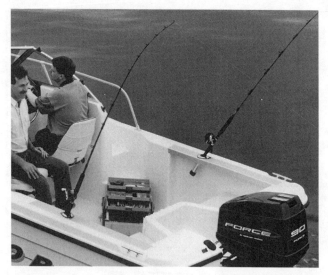

This Bayliner 1802 Trophy walkaround console boat features dual rod holders on the gunwales. Such holders keep the rods out of the way when not fishing, and can be used for trolling, as these anglers are doing.

as well. And it serves as an extra seat.) Aftermarket features, such as rod racks and livewells, are available from a number of manufacturers and offer the boat fisherman a choice of features as well as a method of spreading out the cost of an outfitted boat over a few years. We'll cover some of these accessories in more detail in Chapter 6.

2

FISHING BOAT TYPES

Boat styles have changed considerably over the years, especially in recent times. Specialization has taken over the boat industry in a big way, which is directly reflected in craft designed for fishing that are now on the market.

Again, though, a boat needn't be a specialized, expensive craft in order for one to take it fishing. As a matter of fact, for many years freshwater fishermen had absolutely no problem catching fish from boats that were designed for all-around use. These "utility boats" are still in evidence today, with thousands of anglers using them to catch fish in ponds and lakes, creeks, and rivers. Let's examine these first.

SKIFFS/UTILITY BOATS

For our purposes, this category of boats includes all those small (eight to sixteen feet or so) open boats that were designed for general use. They

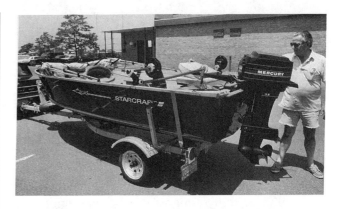

This 14½-foot aluminum Starcraft utility boat is fully tricked out for this angler's style of fishing: dual downriggers, adjustable and removable rod holders, adjustable and removable seats with seat backs, and folding canopy for sunny days on the water.

go by a number of names, but there is so much crossover of styles among them that, for our purposes, it is pointless to hang a name on each. For example, a *dinghy* is a very small utility boat, usually with a pointed bow and square stern. A *pram*, on the other hand, is a very small utility boat, usually with a squared-off bow and stern. But you wouldn't be incorrect in calling either one a *rowboat*, because both dinghies and prams have oarlocks, and so can be propelled by oars. But the term *rowboat* is usually reserved for a large skiff with a high bow—and a *skiff* looks an awful lot like a rowboat, though some purists may insist that a skiff is narrower. And *cartopper* is another often-used boat description—but if you can carry your dinghy, or pram, or rowboat, or skiff on top of your vehicle, then which term is correct?

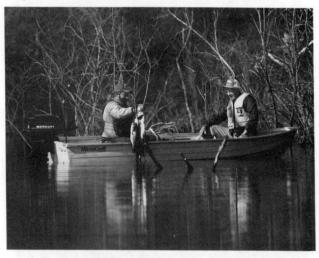

Utility boats offer plenty of room for tackle, gear, and fish, and don't need a powerful outboard to move them.

Obviously, it doesn't matter. What *is* important, however, is that numerous boat manufacturers still produce skiff/utility boats, because there is still quite a market for them. They incorporate no features specific to fishing, but their low price, inherent portability, ease of use, and low maintenance make them very attractive to anglers across the country.

Skiff/utility boats come in aluminum and fiberglass. Some wooden boats are still made by small builders, usually to supply a local demand. The problem with wooden boats, of course, is weight. They're not impossible to hoist up onto a car's roof rack, but an aluminum boat of the same design makes the job a cinch by comparison. And wooden boats do require maintenance, most often painting. So the fisherman in the market for a skiff/utility boat should look to fiberglass or aluminum construction, and focus on the latter if mobility on land is important.

Almost all skiff/utility boats can be powered by an outboard motor. The light weight of these boats means that you don't need a lot of horsepower to push them. A twelve-footer, for example, often needs no more than a $7\frac{1}{2}$-horsepower outboard to get around in most waters where that size boat is safe to use. And a 5- or 6-horsepower outboard will still be adequate for the majority of fishing uses.

Many owners of skiff/utility boats, however, don't bother with an outboard, because the waters they fish aren't so large that a set of oars and a little bit of muscle won't get you to where you want to go. Going sans motor has the added attraction of a smaller financial investment to get you out on the water.

One final advantage of skiff/utility boats: a number of waters, especially reservoirs, enforce a horsepower restriction. Many require that boaters use outboards of less than 10 horsepower. Obviously, only a small boat such as a skiff/utility can be adequately powered by such a motor. (Additionally, this is the reason why many outboard manufacturers make motors of 9.9 horsepower. More on this in Chapter 4.)

Most skiff/utility boats on today's market have a pointed bow and a hull with some type of V configuration. Generally, if a utility boat has a flat-bottomed hull and squared-off bow and stern, it is a johnboat.

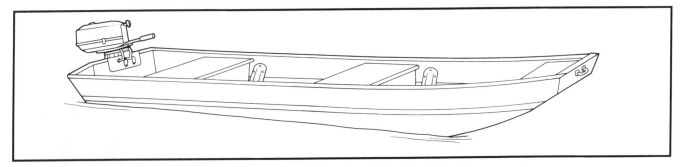

A johnboat, with its flat bottom and minimal displacement, moves easily through the water and is perfect for fishing shallow waters such as a bass pond.

JOHNBOATS

A johnboat is a utility boat with a specific purpose: namely, to navigate shallow water easily. Boats with V hulls obviously are problematic in rivers with numerous shoals and gravel bars, as well as in shallow bass lakes and bream ponds.

The johnboat was developed in the Ozark mountains, specifically for the purpose of floating the shoals-and-rapids streams in that region. The basic design—a flat bottom and square bow—has endured for decades, and has plenty of uses that appeal to the modern fisherman.

A johnboat's flat bottom will skid right over submerged obstructions. This is probably the most important attribute of johnboats, because for all its disadvantages, the johnboat often is the *only* craft that can navigate shallow impoundments, farm ponds, rivers with rocks and blowdowns lying just beneath the surface, and flooded shorelines.

The other major advantage of the johnboat is its ability to carry quite a heavy load for its size. Such a feature—which many fishermen find just as important as its shallow-water ability—is a result of the johnboat's width, or beam, in proportion to its length. The flat bottom floats the johnboat so high that its draft is very shallow, even when jammed to capacity with anglers and equipment.

Johnboats run ten to sixteen feet long, and nearly all of them are made out of aluminum, which allows them entry into the "cartopper" category. Some are so lightweight—a hundred pounds or so—that an angler can load, unload, and launch one alone. And the johnboat's relatively simple design allows manufacturers to produce them inexpensively.

Disadvantages? Johnboats don't handle rough water very well at all, given the flat hull shape. And the low, square bow won't ward off water in a chop. This can translate into anything from an uncomfortably wet ride to a dangerous situation, as the bow can actually help "shovel" water right in if taking a wave head-on. Because of their comparatively primitive design, older-model johnboats can give occupants quite a pounding, even in a relatively mild blow, and can be tippy as well. And the flat hull does not help a rower keep a straight course, often yawing from side to side in a wind.

But outboard motors take well to johnboats, as their shallow-draft hulls move through the water easily with very little horsepower. This presents another savings to the johnboat buyer, who won't need as large an outboard as for a V-hull utility boat of the same size. Even a drop in just one or two horses can mean a price reduction of several hundred dollars.

The johnboat is not the perfect all-around boat, but it is ideal for many purposes and the only choice for a few of them.

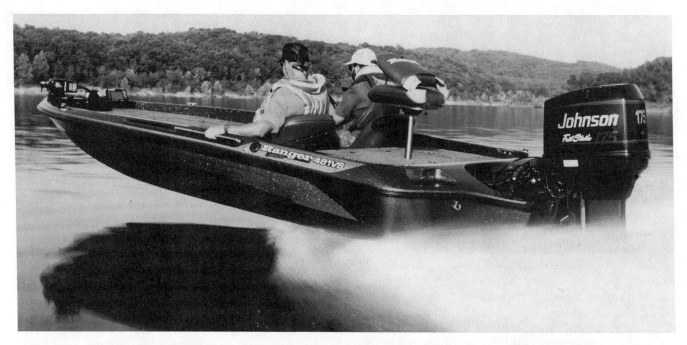

A bass boat under way. This (the 461VS Comanche from Ranger Boats) and many other bass boats are designed to ride only on the rear "pad" upon reaching planing speed.

BASS BOATS

Throughout the South and parts of the Midwest are hundreds of large lakes and man-made impoundments where the largemouth bass is the primary gamefish species. Back in the 1960s, the allure of largemouth bass fishing spread like influenza, due in no small part to the advent of the Bass Anglers Sportsman Society (BASS), an organization that exists to this day. BASS organized and promoted bass-fishing tournaments with large cash prizes for the heaviest catches, and the outdoor press would tout the results of these contests.

The quarry of tournament fishermen were huge largemouths—"hawgs"—in Alabama, Georgia, Florida, and other states that experience mild winters and hence have a long "growing season" for largemouths. The majority of the waters are vast in size, often consisting of a lowland or valley flooded by the damming of rivers in the region. The reservoirs are deep in the middle areas, but the lake arms and backwaters and elbows, which resulted from the flooding, can be shallow.

The bass fishing then was (and, thanks to the advent of catch-and-release, still is) very good—if the angler could find the fish. What was needed was a boat-and-motor combination small enough to be trailerable but powerful enough to move from place to place on these expansive waters. It had to have a hull that could rise up on plane quickly, but still provide reasonable stability. And it had to be comfortable enough to stay in all day, if that's what it took to find the bass.

The bass boat was born.

The metamorphosis of the bass boat, from the first models to today's rigs, isn't as important as the recognition that bass boats aren't for the occasional, or even the average, fisherman. They are not designed for use in small rivers and streams, and are not capable of handling extremely rough water. And they are not inexpensive. But if you have your eye on fishing big, relatively calm waters—and if you're willing to make a fairly hefty cash investment—then a bass boat may be for you.

The first bass boats were made of plywood and looked like johnboats. Most bass boats today are fiberglass, though a few manufacturers have come out with aluminum models. The hulls are usually a sharp V shape at the bow, tapering to a flat area or "pad" near the stern, on which the boat rides when up on plane. They average sixteen to a bit over twenty feet long, and have a steering console with remote power controls. They are generally powered by powerful outboard motors—a 200-horsepower outboard on a twenty-footer is not a rarity—and have built-in fuel tanks. The overall shape of the craft is streamlined, with manufacturers engineering a myriad of hydrodynamic—and aerodynamic—designs to increase the boat's speed. Most are outfitted with comfortable padded seats that are meant for use when under power, not when fishing. Amenities such as rod storage holders, pedestal seats, livewells, engine gauges, and fishing electronics are either standard or optional.

Bass boats are extremely fast (some approach one hundred miles per hour), very stable at rest, comfortable to fish in, fuel-efficient when used in the waters they were designed for, and a heck of a lot of fun to operate and ride in. But they are specialized craft, and probably not the best choice for an angler's very first boat unless he or she can't live without one.

MULTISPECIES BOATS

This is a recently coined term for a craft that, through years of modification and finessing by numerous manufacturers, is designed for freshwater fishermen across the United States.

The multispecies boat is basically a utility boat with all the bells and whistles of a modern bass boat. The primary difference is in the hull shape: multispecies boats usually have a deep-V hull, to enable their use in all water conditions, including big waters that can become choppy. They are designed to handle powerful outboards, but not to provide the very high speed of bass boats. The multis also have a generally "open" aspect, affirming their utility-boat ancestry—no bulky structures to impede anglers moving about the boat or casting to fish.

A predecessor or companion of the multispecies boat, depending on the maker of the craft, is the *walleye* boat. (Many manufacturers still label their multispecies boats as such.) The walleye boat has its origins in the midwestern United States, where the walleye is one of if not the most sought-after species among anglers. Fishermen there needed a craft that was large enough for comfortable fishing, small enough to easily trailer to various lakes and rivers, with a hull that would provide stability and protection in rough water—the "walleye chop" that is usually considered conducive to good fishing. Also necessary were features such as remote steering and throttle, built-in fuel tanks, carpeted flooring, baitwells, livewells, pedestal seats, tackle storage, and easy adaptability to fishing electronics such as sonar units.

This functional design resulted in a craft that is perfect for fishing in waters that are home to fish other than walleyes, and thus has appeal to anglers other than walleye fishermen.

Numerous manufacturers design all manner of multispecies boats, both aluminum and fiberglass. They average sixteen to eighteen feet in length,

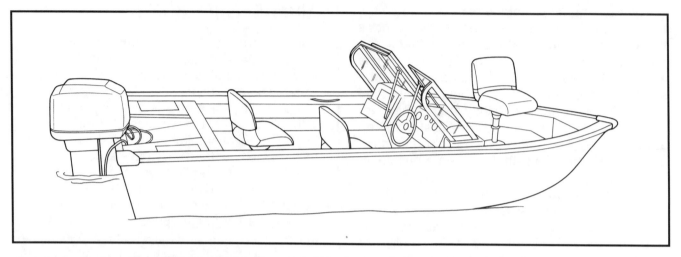

A good example of a multispecies boat: console with seats, built-in electronics, windshield, fairly powerful outboard—but with a hull that can handle rough water if the situation arises.

and take outboards up to 150 horsepower (though many do just fine with motors of less than 100 hp). They trailer very easily, and extra features may be added to these boats whenever the owner has the inclination.

Multispecies boats fit the needs of thousands of anglers. Constant updating and redesigning by manufacturers give the prospective boat buyer a plethora of choices. Multi boats, a relatively recent phenomenon, are here to stay.

CONSOLE BOATS

Here we enter the realm of the big-water boats, those designed for use in large lakes, reservoirs, and rivers. Their deep draft prohibits their use in shallow waters, and often such boats are way too overpowered for small waters.

For our uses in this book, the term *console boat* will encompass a number of various styles of craft. Minimum size for a console boat is about sixteen feet. Most are fiberglass, though some are constructed of aluminum. Most of them incorporate features for fishermen: livewells, fish boxes, rod storage.

The common feature among them is a console, which at minimum consists of a steering wheel, a throttle control, and engine gauges. Those are the basic components; numerous other controls (such as a depthfinder) and devices (a windshield) may be placed on the console.

The reason for a console is quite simple: boats that require a motor powerful enough to safely push them around a large body of water cannot be easily operated directly from a tiller.

Some console boats are powered by an outboard motor, or even a pair of them. This offers the obvious advantage of extra power, as well as a safety precaution should one outboard quit. Others have a stern-drive (inboard/outboard, or I/O) motor pushing them (see Chapter 4). Motors of 50 to 225 horsepower are necessary.

The following are the commonly accepted

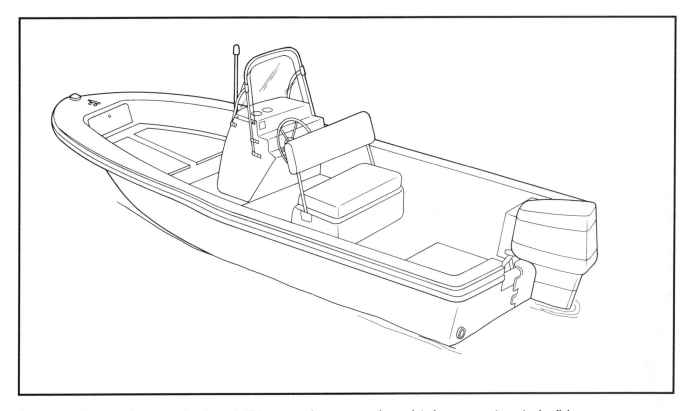

Center-console boats offer many advantages to fishermen, primary among them a lot of open space to cast, play fish, and keep gear accessible.

terms for the various styles of console boats appropriate for fishing in freshwater (again keeping to our maximums of 26 feet in length and 8½ feet in width, or beam):

Center Consoles

This is an ideal style of craft for many anglers because the console is situated directly in the center of the deck, with room to walk past on the left and right (port and starboard). Some center consoles have one or two seats for the operator and another person; others have a "leaning post" situated where seats would be placed. As there is no other structure on the deck, anglers are free to move about the entire craft to cast, drop lines, or play a fish. More tackle and equipment may be carried as well, as the spartan layout allows full use of the deck area.

Disadvantages of a center console: minimal protection from wind and spray, other than that provided by the console itself. Except for storage boxes built into the hull, there is no place to protect gear from exposure to the elements.

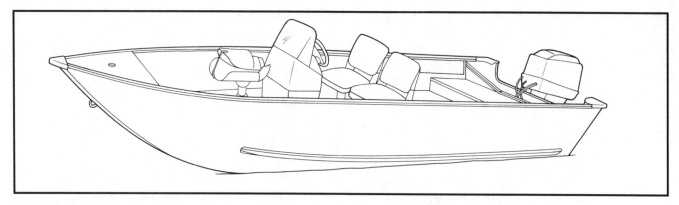

Side consoles free up one whole side of the boat, which eases certain angling methods such as drift-fishing.

Side Consoles

As its name implies, the side-console boat has the console placed to one side of the deck, either port or starboard, with a seat for the operator. Some side consoles offer a seat placed backward directly behind the operator's seat (called a back-to-back seat). Such a design frees up the entire other side of the craft. The side console is advantageous

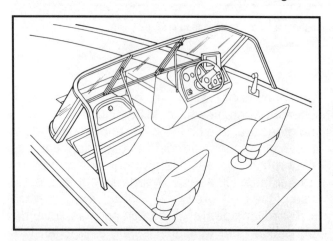

The twin-console or walkthrough boat offers protection and seating comfort for two anglers. Some twin consoles, such as Ranger's 692VS Fisherman, offer a removable windshield that can be inserted between the console windshields to provide additional protection from wind and spray.

for certain fishing applications, such as when drifting with the wind or current. All anglers aboard can line up on the free side of the boat and fish comfortably.

Disadvantages: As with the center console, the side console offers minimal protection from wind and spray. The operator obtains some shelter from the console itself (especially if there is a windshield), but other occupants and gear are exposed.

Twin Consoles

The twin, or dual, console is a side console with another noncontrol console across from it. Both the boat operator and at least one passenger then have comfortable and protected seats. If dual back-to-back seats are in place, then the operator and three passengers are offered some degree of protection.

Many twin consoles have a separate windshield for each console. Such an arrangement may be called a *walkthrough*, because anglers can pass between the consoles to reach the bow. A number of twin consoles today offer the option of a windshield that fits between the two consoles' windshields, thereby creating one complete windshield from port to starboard. This allows the operator to insert the windshield when running, to protect all aboard from wind and spray, and to remove it when fishing, to allow unimpeded access to the bow.

Disadvantage: what is gained in shelter is lost in free deck space. But such a sacrifice is well worth it to anglers who fish in rough waters.

Walkarounds

The walkaround boat features a raised console that extends to the bow and almost to the port and starboard sides. This allows occupants reasonable access to the bow, as well as some ability to move about the entire boat to cast or play a fish. Below the console is a berth for storage.

Some walkaround berths contain a head (toilet) and/or bunks for resting.

The raised console on a walkaround boat provides good protection from water and wind, and many anglers find a berth very practical, especially those who want a place in which to rest comfortably, or even stay overnight, without having to leave the boat.

Disadvantages: again, more structure equates with less roominess for fishing. And not all walkarounds allow easy access to the bow: the passage is usually very narrow, and people must hold on to a rail to keep their balance when walking to the bow.

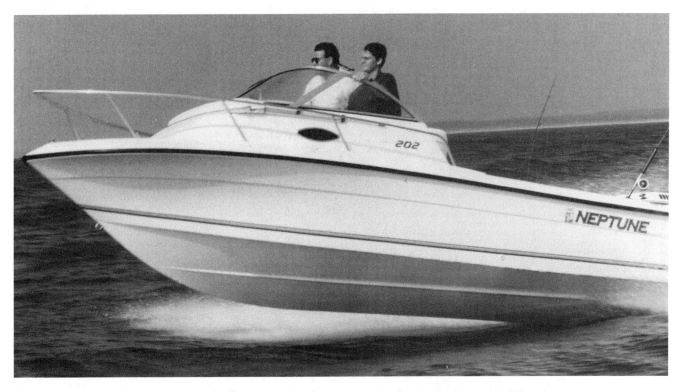

The walkaround boat allows anglers reasonable access to the bow while offering a great degree of protection. Some walkarounds, such as this Neptune 202 from Sunbird, also have a cabin large enough to bunk in, though most cabins on this type of boat offer a very limited amount of space.

17

Cuddy Cabins

Similar to a walkaround, the cuddy cabin features a raised console with berth beneath, except there is no easy passage to the bow from the cockpit. The gain is a larger berth, or cuddy.

The obvious disadvantage to cuddy cabins is the small amount of space available to the angler; basically fishing is possible only from the console rearward. For this reason cuddy cabins are not the best choice for fishing boats—but, for fishermen who intend to use their boats for other recreational pursuits such as waterskiing, the cuddy makes perfect sense. It offers plenty of storage space, room to sleep, and good protection from wind and water.

Keep in mind that numerous other boat styles exist, but they are not covered here because they are not suitable freshwater fishing craft. Also, the boat styles that are discussed here are not rigidly conformed to by boat manufacturers. Some companies make boats that combine two styles, such as a *walkaround cuddy*.

A new type of fishing boat design apparently is aimed at the recreational boater who fishes, or possibly the fisherman who boats recreationally.

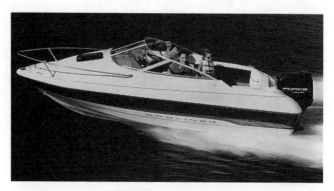

A true cuddy-cabin boat does not offer a comfortable fishing platform on the bow but does contain a sizable berth—large enough to sleep in overnight. This cuddy cabin, the 1702 Capri LS from Bayliner, has a narrow transom, which makes fishing easier.

These are the "fish/sport" or "fish/ski" boats, which combine the amenities of recreational boats—such as ample seating arrangements—along with fishing features, like fish boxes and livewells. Obviously a family of five would not find much comfort on, say, a center console with no seats that doesn't block spray, so these designs make sense and have earned a place in the fishing boat market.

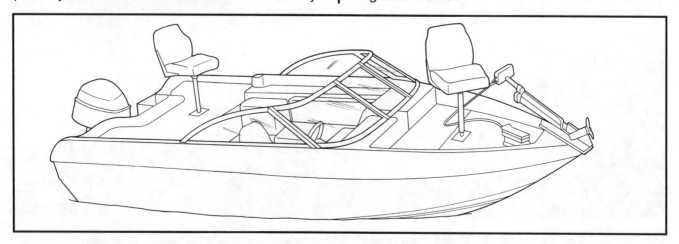

New on the market are combination "fish/ski" boats. With features dedicated to both anglers and waterskiers, these dual-purpose craft appeal to anglers who have family or friends who don't fish.

Flats Boats for Freshwater

Having its origins in the Caribbean, and especially known in the United States as the boat to fish the Florida flats for tarpon, bonefish, and permit, the flats boat is becoming popular in other areas of the country. Although many anglers are discovering the attributes of the flats boat for use in saltwater on both the Atlantic and Gulf coasts, its use is certainly not limited to the brine.

The flats boat was first built to provide anglers with a very fast method of traveling through shallow waters to distant locations. Once there, the angler or boat operator must be able to quickly and easily pole the boat through promising flats, visually searching for gamefish. Also, the angler needs a fairly long, wide, and stable platform from which to cast to and eventually play powerful fish on light tackle.

The growth of fly-fishing is probably connected to the growth of flats boats, as these craft provide a perfect platform for fly-casting maneuverability. Whether casting to a Florida bonefish or a New York bluefish, the fly fisherman must keep large amounts of fly line loose at his feet and be able to turn and cast to a fish quickly.

These flats boats are perfectly adaptable to freshwater fishing because they are fast, highly maneuverable, extremely comfortable and roomy, and are designed with a number of fishing amenities such as rod lockers, livewells, and tackle storage compartments. Actually, many flats boats bear striking resemblances to bass boats, in that they are streamlined craft powered by high-horsepower outboards. Hull shapes vary, but typically flatten out at the stern from a V-shaped bow. But flats boats are relatively wide for their length, which provides good stability even in a chop.

One drawback to most flats boats is a lack of occupant protection from wind and water. Though most flats boats have steering consoles, for the most part they are low and lack windshields. Still, they are well-designed fishing machines and excel at a number of freshwater fishing applications, such as big-lake fly-fishing in warm-weather areas.

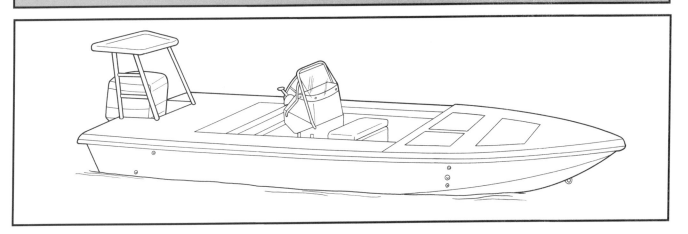

Flats boats aren't just for saltwater. This 2020 Flatsmaster from Action Craft is perfect for fly-fishing in large lakes because the flat, open bow allows plenty of casting room, is easy to balance on, and has no obstructions that loose fly line can snag on.

3

ALTERNATIVE CRAFT

Some fishing situations require special craft to put anglers in the best position to catch fish. Other times, a certain type of boat allows an angler to fish otherwise unattainable waters. Finally, some boats are built specifically for people who have very limited storage space at home.

These are the alternative craft: canoes, inflatable boats, pontoon boats, and take-down boats. All have specific angling functions, and one of them may be the best choice for you either as a primary boat, or as a backup.

CANOES

For the ultimate combination of carrying capacity, light weight, easy storage, and durability, a canoe is hard to beat. Modern canoes are made of light-weight aluminum, fiberglass, or Kevlar, with aluminum the most predominant. One sixteen-foot aluminum canoe—which is about average size—has a person-weight capacity of 565 pounds, yet

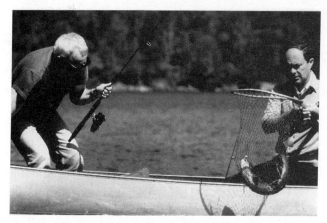

Canoes work well on large waters as well as small ones, as these lake trout anglers found out.

weighs only 69 pounds. Two people can easily carry such a craft to wooded streams and back-woods ponds without much strain, and fish waters that no other boat owners could even think about.

Canoes are also appropriate for fishing rock-studded streams, as their streamlined shape allows for easy maneuvering through narrow passages. One sweep of a paddle will alter the canoe's course, thereby making easy work of avoiding hazards. And when a silent approach is necessary—such as slipping up on the weedy shallows of a bass pond—the canoe is the perfect choice.

Obviously canoes are not the ultimate all-around fishing craft. They are not very stable, and certainly are not suitable for fishing large bodies of water. Canoes also are not the most comfortable of craft, at least when compared with boats with cushioned seats. They don't offer a lot of elbow room—people who try to stand up in a canoe often wind up wet.

The keel of a canoe will dictate its intended use. A standard keel is meant for still waters and general canoeing in relatively smooth rivers. The standard keel makes for easy paddling, as it helps keep the canoe "on track," or on a steady course. A shallow keel or no keel at all makes for smoother rides over rocks and other obstructions in shallow water, and is also more responsive to the paddle. Canoe manufacturers all have their own keel types, but basically the choice boils down to stability or maneuverability. Most anglers would be wise to choose stability over responsiveness.

Two basic designs of canoes are the double-ender and the square stern. The double-ender has a pointed bow and stern. It is the classic canoe shape, streamlined and wind resistant and able to move backward as easily as forward. The square stern is designed solely for the addition of an outboard motor to the canoe, though side-mount motor brackets are available to fit outboards to double-enders.

A number of options available for canoes benefit their use for fishing. A rowing bracket, for example, allows the canoeing fisherman to row his canoe rather than paddle it. Solo fishermen

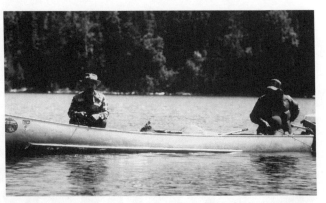

Square-stern canoes are made for outboard power. Double-end canoes can be fitted with a bracket to take outboards as well.

on lakes find such a device makes getting around much easier. Sponsons, which are flotation devices that clamp on to the canoe's gunwales, provide additional balance and stability.

Canoes are so lightweight that almost any vehicle can carry one easily and safely with the addition of a roof rack. They also store well, at any angle, and do not take up much room. Some owners keep their canoes roped to a garage or basement ceiling during the off-season. Add to all this a low purchase price and the low or zero maintenance involved, and the canoe turns out to be the perfect small-water craft for anglers who don't require many amenities.

INFLATABLES

Buoyancy and portability are the key features of the inflatable boat. Many modern inflatables come with a rigid hull and deck, which are the best choices for fishermen for security and stability (and because fish hooks sometimes penetrate objects other than fish). Inflatables can be outfitted with outboard motors, and their carrying capacity is surprisingly high: the Quicksilver Rigid-Hull Inflatable, which measures ten feet nine inches, can handle a total of 1,500 pounds of anglers, motor, and gear.

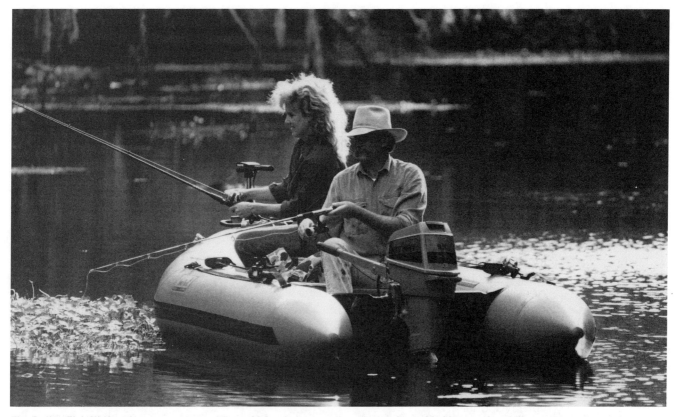

The Zodiac Fish N' Hunt features a plywood floor, 20-horsepower outboard capacity, rod holders, and a trolling motor mount.

Air chambers on inflatables are typically separated, which provides stability (in case of uneven inflation) and safety. Long gone are the days of "rubber boats." Skins of modern inflatables are made of rugged, abrasion-resistant PVC, nylon, and/or polyester, which aren't severely affected by sunlight.

Inflatables float incredibly well, which is understandable considering that they're filled with air. This is why whitewater specialists find inflatables the best craft going for their needs. Inflatables manage to stay upright when being tossed around the haystacks and into the holes, even when carrying a heavy load.

As with canoes, inflatables are worth consider-

ation by anglers with limited home storage space. Many inflatables—rigid hull included—fold down into a container small enough to fit into the trunk of a compact car. Anglers who live in an apartment or condominium—people who would never even consider boat ownership—can keep an inflatable in a closet.

Zodiac, one of the oldest names in inflatable craft, makes a model specifically designed for sportsmen. Called the Fish N' Hunt, the craft has a full-length segmented plywood floor and separate air chambers that will keep the boat afloat even with a couple of them deflated. The $12\frac{1}{2}$-foot model is olive green and has a weight capacity of 1,190 pounds, equivalent to five or six people.

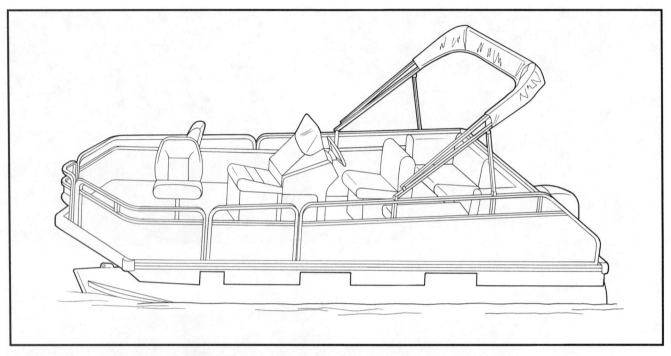

Pontoon boats are definitely viable fishing craft. This Sun Tracker Bass Buggy measures eighteen feet long and eight feet wide and can safely hold up to seven people.

The boat can take up to a 20-horsepower outboard mounted in a unique motor well. Standard equipment includes rod holders and a trolling motor mount on the bow. When disassembled, the whole craft—including motor and accessories—will fit into the back of a station wagon. This is a craft definitely worth considering by anglers who lack storage space.

PONTOON BOATS

Leisure time may or may not have increased in the United States, but appreciation of it has certainly grown. This appears to be one reason for the tremendous popularity of the pontoon boat—and may explain why it is sometimes referred to as a "party barge."

The pontoon boat is basically a large aluminum or fiberglass motorized raft with console control, a lot of deck space, and a comfortable seating arrangement. The flotation system consists of twin aluminum pontoons or fiberglass sponsons with separate chambers, a safety precaution in the event of puncture. The boats themselves are wide—average beam is eight feet—and range from eighteen to twenty-six feet in length.

Some plain-Jane models come with nothing but seats and a console. But an incredible array of upgrades and features on pricier models make these some of the most luxurious small craft afloat: stereo sound systems, carpet, tables, galley with sink, toilet, shower, gas grill, pull-out sleep sofas, vinyl enclosures with windows.

So what attraction do pontoon boats have for fishermen?

They are not as cumbersome as they appear. The Sun Tracker Party Express twenty-four footer, for example, has a draft of only ten inches. The package model comes with an outboard of only 90 horsepower—a comparatively small and inexpensive-to-operate motor—yet is powerful enough to tow a waterskier. So with these attributes alone fishermen have a trailerable boat that can reach impressive speeds without undue cost, yet still get around the shallows if necessary.

Additionally, a few pontoon models are geared specifically for fishermen. Features such as pedestal seats, livewells, coolers, rod holders, and extra storage space are available on some makes.

The result is versatility. An angler who could not justify the expense of a fully outfitted bass boat may find a pontoon boat perfectly logical, as his nonfishing friends and/or family will be able to enjoy it for waterskiing, swimming, or just cruising. Even an eighteen-foot pontoon will hold seven people easily, with room and comfort enough to stay on the water all day. Pontoons incorporate a number of safety features, such as high rails all around the craft, so children can be brought aboard with no undue worry.

Pontoon boats are far from the ideal fishing craft, but they do fulfill a number of angling needs. And they just may be the perfect all-around craft for family recreation.

PORTABLE BOATS

This is somewhat a misnomer because so many small boats are, of course, portable. But it has become the accepted industry term for a boat that is portable in the sense that it folds into flat sections, much like a toy balsawood airplane.

But these are far from toys. The Porta-Bote Genesis III, for example, is constructed of tough polypropylene, measures twelve feet in length when assembled, can hold four people, and takes up to a 7-horsepower outboard. Without seats it weighs sixty-nine pounds and folds down into a package eleven feet long, but only two feet wide and four inches thick—very practical for anglers who have to carry their boat long distances to launch it, such as on remote waters.

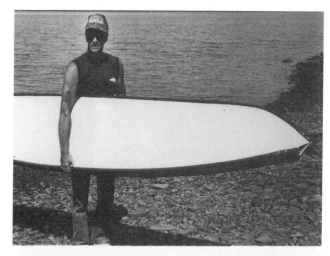

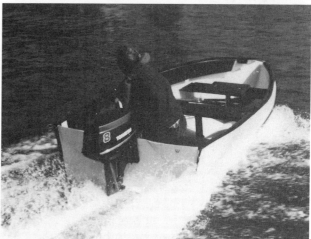

The Porta-Bote Genesis III: a twelve-foot utility boat that actually folds into a package eleven feet long, two feet wide, and four inches thick.

4

MOTORS

Unless you like to row, you'll need something to move your craft from launching ramp to fishing area and back again.

The good news is that boat-motor technology has caught up with some of the engineering advancements of the age. This was not always the case. For many years, outboards and stern drives did not show any advancements or improvements in efficiency, maintenance, power, and weight. Today's boat motors reflect state-of-the-art design in such things as fuel and ignition systems, metal strength, and noncorrosive composites.

The bad news, or at least the cost of such improvements, is just that—the cost. Fortunately the majority of modern boat motors are extremely reliable and will yield top performance for many years, so paying the price for a good motor can be considered an investment toward satisfying and trouble-free fishing. The adage "you get what

you pay for" is never more true than when purchasing a boat motor.

But the prospective boat owner must be sure that the motor bought is the one needed. A motor that runs like a top does little good if it's the wrong choice for the boat it's pushing.

BOAT/MOTOR PACKAGES

One easy way to avoid this problem is to buy your boat and motor as a package. This is not a new idea. Boat dealers have been selling boat/motor combinations for years. However, agreements between boat companies and motor companies (as well as arrangements made by corporations that own both boat divisions and motor divisions) have resulted in boat/motor combination packages that are perfectly compatible—and sometimes just plain perfect. The price of the package usually reflects some financial incentive by the company or companies involved—the package is

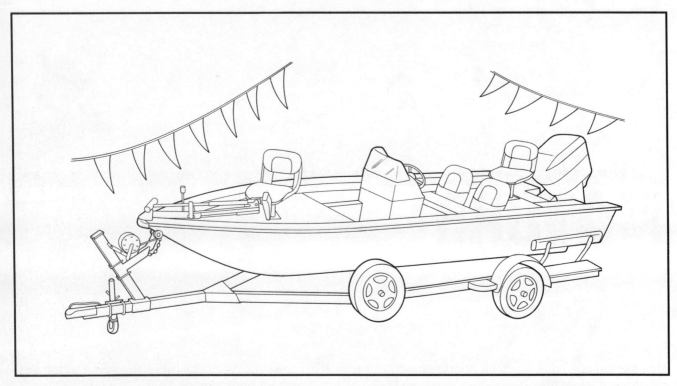

Many boat manufacturers as well as boat dealers sell boat and motor (and trailer) packages, relieving the prospective buyer of additional shopping and researching.

often cheaper than buying the boat and a similar but different make of motor separately.

Some companies will offer different motor package options for the same boat, with the most inexpensive package including the lowest horsepower motor. This is where you'll have to figure how much power you'll need, which will involve the weight of people and gear you will usually have on board, and the type of water you plan on fishing. Running a powerful motor at three-quarters throttle is more efficient than running a less powerful motor at full throttle, so also try to figure how much long-distance cruising you'll be doing. More on this later.

OUTBOARDS

The majority of freshwater fishing boats are powered by outboard motors. Outboards offer many advantages and usually are the only choice in power anyway. Ranging in size from mini motors of less than 1 horsepower to behemoth 300-horsepower V-8s, outboards produce a lot of power for their weight. And because outboards are mounted off the stern, more free space is available on board the boat. Smaller outboards can be easily removed from the boat and brought indoors for off-season storage and/or maintenance.

Outboards are easily trimmed (adjusting the angle of the propeller and shaft in relation to the boat) for increased performance and efficiency. This can be done manually, by moving an adjustment bar beneath the engine, or electronically on models equipped with power trim.

If you want to or have to buy the outboard separately from your boat, the first decision to make concerns the size. The place to start is the National Marine Manufacturers Association rating and capacity plate that is attached to your boat, usually on the inside of the transom. In addition to other statistics about the boat, the plate will list the maximum recommended horsepower of outboard motor to use on that craft. (Exceeding that rating is dangerous because as horsepower increases, so does the size of the outboard. Overweighing a boat can easily lead to a mishap.)

The largest motor possible on the boat is not always the best choice. The first reason is price: again, as horsepower increases, so does cost. There's no point spending extra money on horsepower that you will never use. Second, the type of hull on your boat may provide satisfactory performance with a less powerful motor. For instance, a modified-V hull needs less horsepower to get on plane than does a deep-V hull, because there's less boat to lift out of the water on the modified V.

So if you want to go lower than maximum, how low should you go? Some experts recommend using the 25:1 ratio: for every 25 pounds of gross boat weight (boat, motor, people, gear), the boat needs 1 horsepower. If you figure your boat will weigh 1,000 pounds fully loaded, you'll need about a 40-horsepower motor. This figure may be close to or as high as the maximum recommended horsepower on your rating plate.

Other industry experts recommend a simpler formula. That is to go with an outboard that produces 75 percent of the maximum horsepower listed on the rating plate. Such a motor size should power the boat more than adequately in

just about all situations. And choosing an outboard that is 35 to 45 percent less than the maximum will probably be satisfactory.

Again, keep in mind the efficiency rule: a large motor at three-quarters throttle uses less gas than a smaller motor at full throttle.

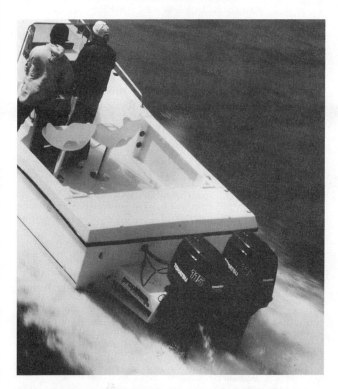

Some anglers, especially those who fish large waters far offshore, prefer two outboards of medium horsepower for the boat instead of one high-horsepower motor.

DOUBLING UP

Many larger fishing boats have the capacity to handle two outboards. There are good reasons for doing so, other than the apparent and seemingly not-so-important one of increased speed.

Mechanical difficulties will occur, no matter how much care you give an outboard. Even a sparkling new outboard with less than one hour's running time could run into floating timber and break a prop blade. If you're on an average-size lake, your only worries might be a sore shoulder from paddling your way to shore or another boat and the ensuing repair bill.

But if you're caught way offshore on a huge reservoir, or on one of the Great Lakes, you're in serious trouble. For starters, the towing bill can be astronomical. And let's not even consider the possibility of a bad storm brewing at that time.

The chances of two motors breaking down at exactly the same time are very low. If one outboard should break down, you could make your way back with the other.

OUTBOARDS OF 15 HORSEPOWER AND LESS

These are the smallest outboards on the market and are perfect for pushing small skiffs, utility boats, and johnboats. Those of 5 horsepower or less excel as power for canoes and inflatables.

Practically all of these outboards are operated via a combination tiller/throttle, which permits the operator to steer the boat and increase or reduce power simultaneously. A separate control allows shifting from a drive position to neutral (not all motors in this class have a reverse gear). Obviously the operator must sit in the stern of the boat and maintain constant contact with the tiller when under way.

Many of these small outboards, especially the lower-horsepower versions, have a built-in fuel tank. Others come with a remote tank and must be connected via a fuel line. In either case, modern motors of this size are marvelously efficient and very lightweight. Even the most powerful outboard in this class can be carried without strain: the Mercury 15-horsepower two-stroke weighs only seventy-one pounds.

The starting mechanism on most of these small outboards is a built-in rope-pull (often termed

Because a number of waters across the country are restricted to boats with outboards of less than 10 horsepower, the 9.9 makes sense. This Evinrude is a four-stroke.

Dressed to the Nines

Assigning a 9.9-horsepower designation to an outboard may not appear logical. Why not make it 10? The reason is that a number of lakes and impoundments across the country enforce a "less than 10" regulation—that is, all motors on boats must be of less than 10 horsepower. Such a rule effectively prohibits large craft from using the lake, which results in smaller wakes from passing craft, reduced noise levels, easier going for those in non-motorized craft, and, theoretically, a more pleasant aspect. This rule does make sense on relatively small bodies of water near highly populated areas. And, happily, it keeps waterskiers away.

"manual start") similar to that on a lawn mower. Electric start is available on some, but a battery then becomes necessary. The engines themselves are typically two-cylinders, and are two-stroke in design, which means that oil must be premixed with gasoline.

Some remote tanks on these (and larger) outboards mix the oil and gasoline automatically. The operator simply fills the gasoline reservoir and the oil reservoir on the remote tank and hooks up the fuel line to the outboard. There is then no need to tediously measure out the proper amounts of oil and gasoline each time a tank needs refilling.

OUTBOARDS FROM 20 TO 70 HORSEPOWER

This group of outboards displays transitions in a number of areas. Weight of the motors takes a leap—they range from a bit over 100 pounds for the compact 20-horsepower kickers to around 250 pounds for the big 70-horsepower models. As a result, they are not as portable as their lower-horsepower kin, but they can still be removed from a boat with a little effort (and help) and stored or tuned indoors.

The number of cylinders increases as well. The lower-power motors in this group have two, the higher ones have three. Mercury offers a 40-horsepower model with four cylinders.

Electric start is either optional or standard on almost all motors in this class. Many are available in either tiller steer, for open craft, or remote-control models for console boats. Lower-power versions have one carburetor; higher-power ones have two. Advanced fuel-induction systems are common as well. Power (electronic) trim is optional on many.

Automatic oil injection is also an important feature on these larger outboards. Because more horsepower means more fuel consumption, pre-mixing gas and oil can become a chore. Auto oil injection, either standard or optional on this size of motors, eliminates it.

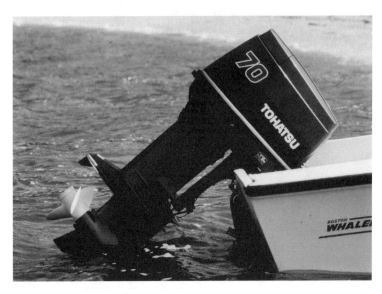

Outboards in the 20- to 70-horsepower category are transitional: some can be carried easily, some cannot; and a number of features are either standard or optional, such as electric start, tiller steer, and certain fuel-induction systems.

Long Shaft or Short?

Shaft length becomes an important consideration with the higher-power outboards, because the styles of boats that take these larger outboards vary widely. (Lower-horsepower outboards are available in a range of shaft lengths as well, but the long-shaft models are used primarily as motorized power for sailboats and as auxiliary power for larger boats.)

The proper shaft length depends on the height of the boat's transom. For example, standard shaft lengths for small- to medium-sized boats are fifteen inches for short shaft, twenty inches for long shaft. The transom itself should, *but does not always*, determine the shaft length to use. The rule of thumb is for the outboard's antiventilation plate, which is the horizontal protrusion above the propeller, to be even with the bottom of the boat.

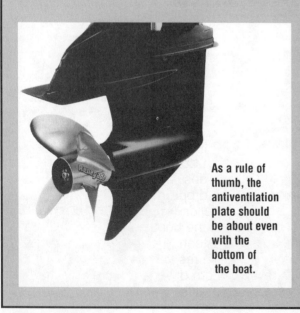

As a rule of thumb, the antiventilation plate should be about even with the bottom of the boat.

OUTBOARDS FROM 75 HORSEPOWER UP

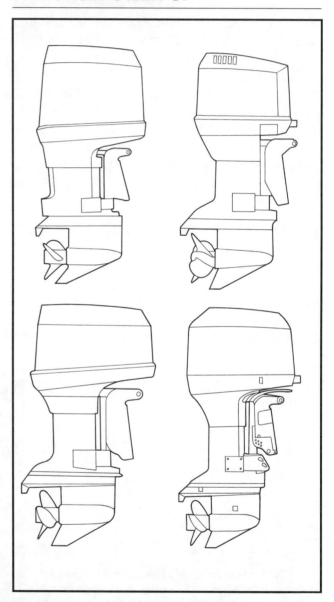

Modern outboards more powerful than 75 horsepower can feature automatic fuel injection, automatic oil injection, and power tilt and trim.

These are the outboards that, because of their size and weight, become practically permanent fixtures on boats. Outboards in this category are removable, of course, but not at all portable.

Although this group encompasses an extremely wide range of horsepower, most of the motors have features unique to their class. Engines are large: three cylinders minimum, growing to V-4, V-6, and finally V-8 in some manufacturers' 250- to 300-horsepower models. With a very few exceptions in the lower-horsepower range, all are steered via remote control, meaning they are for use in boats with a steering console—bass boats, some multispecies boats, and console boats.

Many other features that are optional or not available on outboards in the two smaller classes become standard on many of these motors: electric start (which also requires an alternator system), automatic oil injection, power tilt and trim. Some makers offer electronic fuel injection on their big models.

These large motors are highly engineered and thus extremely expensive. Manufacturers compete keenly for business, and choosing one model over another can be difficult and frustrating. If you haven't decided on a specific boat dealer to buy from, contact the various outboard manufacturers (listed in the appendix at the back of this book) and ask for catalogs and other related literature. If you want to invest plenty of time before you make your decision, attend a boat show in your area and speak to representatives of outboard manufacturers concerning your needs.

Shopping for an outboard in this size class, especially the 220-horsepower-and-up models, is not dissimilar to shopping for a car or truck. Take your time, study the catalogs, become familiar with specifications and warranties, and talk to experienced owners.

Counterrotation

Many large outboards can be ordered with counterrotation, which means that the propeller shaft turns in the opposite direction. This is a useful option to order on an outboard when it will be one of a pair running a boat. Counterrotating propellers ease maneuvering at slow speeds and holding course at high speeds.

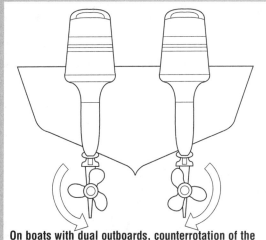

On boats with dual outboards, counterrotation of the propellers improves maneuverability and handling.

STERN DRIVES

The stern drive, or inboard/outboard (I/O), is a boat motor with the engine inside the boat. The lower unit, which consists of the shaft and the propeller, protrudes from the transom above water level and drops down below the surface, where the propeller is located. The lower unit itself turns when the boat is steered. Only a boat with a remote steering console can operate a stern drive, which restricts its use to larger craft.

The typical stern drive is a four-cycle gasoline engine, somewhat similar to those in automo-

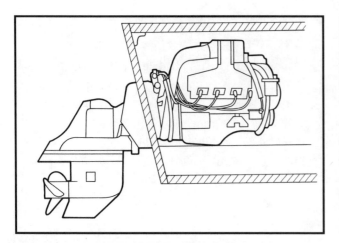

Stern drives, or inboard/outboards, are quieter and more fuel efficient than outboards.

biles, and generally is a power option for large craft. It has a number of advantages over outboards.

Stern drives, with their four-cycle engines, are naturally stingier on gas than are two-cycle outboards. Four-cycle engines require no mixing of gas and oil, as do two-cycle engines, which unless done exactly according to specifications can result in poor performance at best and major engine damage at worst. Four-cycle engines run quieter than two-cycle engines as well. Because the stern drive's engine is located under a hatch inside the boat, it is protected from waves, wakes, spray, and rain. Fewer exposed parts means less chance of mishaps caused by the elements. Routine maintenance is easier to perform because of easy access to the engine.

However, the relatively high cost of a stern drive does not always pay for itself in reduced fuel expenses. The owner must use the boat extensively to realize any financial gain. And any major mechanical problems will prove much more expensive with a stern drive; just the logistics of separating the engine from the lower unit and removing it from the boat equate with higher

costs. Similarly, upgrading to a higher-horsepower motor is not as easily accomplished.

The stern drive does have some appeal, and many boaters wouldn't own a craft without one. But for the majority of freshwater fishermen who own or are considering buying a boat large enough to take either an outboard or a stern drive, the outboard is most practical.

INBOARDS

The inboard engine, which has no lower unit and has an exposed shaft and rudder as well as propeller, is restricted to use on larger craft that typically are not trailered and are kept in the water for the entire boating season, if not year-round. For this reason alone they probably would never be considered by the average freshwater fisherman interested in owning a boat, but several facts are worth pointing out:

Because the inboard has no turning lower unit, the boat must be steered by a rudder. The propeller is located at the end of a long driveshaft. All these exposed parts limit the craft to deep-water use only and require special trailers and launching facilities.

Inboards, which usually are powered by four-cycle gasoline or diesel engines, are quite economical *for the size of boat they are used for*, but are not worthy of consideration here.

FOUR-CYCLE OUTBOARDS

Considering the economical advantages of a four-cycle engine and the practicalities of an outboard, why don't manufacturers come up with the obvious: a four-cycle outboard?

At least one did, back in the 1950s, but at the time there was no need or desire for one. Two-cycle engines are less complicated to manufacture, have fewer parts, and weigh less than four-cycle engines. Still, the idea caught on in a few regions, but never really took hold.

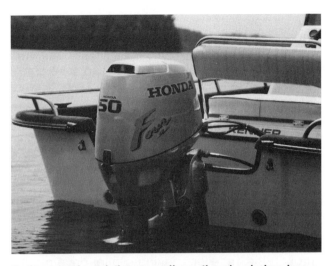

Environmental regulations regarding outboard emissions have resulted in outboard manufacturers' developing four-stroke outboards, such as this Honda 50-horsepower.

But add modern technology and new environmental concern into the equation and the result is a practical and affordable four-cycle outboard. This new family of outboards burns fuel (no mixing of oil and gas!) very efficiently. This yields a cleaner exhaust—much less smoke—and keeps spark plugs from fouling easily. And they are much quieter than two-cycle outboards—not a small consideration when motoring long distances or when sitting within three feet of a 50-horsepower outboard screaming at full throttle. Increasingly strict emission standards and today's stiff prices of petroleum products (not to mention the question of continued easy availability in the future) have encouraged some manufacturers to produce four-cycle outboards.

More parts means a heavier outboard, and more engineering means a higher price tag. But with more and more manufacturers "listening" to consumers, and with good old free-market competitiveness spurring them on, four-cycle outboards will probably earn a permanent place on fishing boats.

JET-DRIVE MOTORS

The jet drive is actually a simple and decades-old concept that, thanks to modern engineering techniques, has exploded in popularity among recreational boaters as well as fishermen. Jet-drive motors, both outboard and stern drive, are now available in relatively lightweight and efficient packages.

Jet drives appeal to fishermen for a number of reasons. First is the lack of a propeller. A jet drive is actually a gasoline-engine-driven water pump.

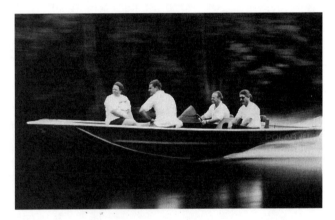

Jet boats, such as this Polar Jet Boat by Polar Kraft, can ride on inches of water and display remarkable handling characteristics.

An impeller (picture a propeller enclosed in a pipe), powered by the engine, draws water in and discharges it at an extremely fast rate. This high-pressure discharge propels the boat forward. The boat is steered by the lower unit turning the direction of the spray. (Reverse is attained by shifting a mechanism in front of the discharge, which throws the flow in the opposite direction.) There is no propeller to become dinged, bent, or broken, and no gearcase seal to become damaged by stray fishing line wrapping around the propeller shaft. Fishermen don't have reason to go overboard very much, but if they do take a spill while the motor is running, the probability of sustaining an injury is much lower.

The second, related benefit of jet motors is their shallow-water capability. The intake on the jet pump has to be just submerged in water to operate; as long as it is below the surface, the boat will move. Therefore, the jet-drive unit does not have to be mounted much lower than the boat's hull—which means that the jet-equipped boat, if it is of the proper configuration, can travel in literally *inches* of water—that is, not much more than the draw of the boat itself. Fishermen in some Midwest states, whose rivers are notable for their prop-eating shoals, have enjoyed this benefit of jet drives for years, though it wasn't until recent times that these motors have been appreciated by many other anglers in the United States.

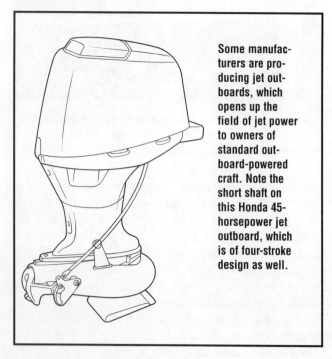

Some manufacturers are producing jet outboards, which opens up the field of jet power to owners of standard outboard-powered craft. Note the short shaft on this Honda 45-horsepower jet outboard, which is of four-stroke design as well.

A jet-powered boat, if it is has a relatively wide and flat hull with well-defined chines, displays astonishing handling capabilities when compared with prop-driven craft. The boat can take sharp turns with ease, even at very high speed. Acceleration occurs with head-snapping swiftness, and coming to a stop is almost as sudden. Such a gymnastic quality may not be critical to many fishermen (discounting tournament anglers and fishermen who frequent rock-studded rivers), but it is an advantage.

Of course, such startling capabilities don't come without some drawbacks. First, jet drives lose about 30 percent of motor horsepower because of the power needed to pump water through the impeller housing. So jet-drive motors aren't as powerful as propeller motors of the same horsepower. Second, the jet pump intake may become clogged with debris, especially when taking off in shallow water. This necessitates stopping and clearing the intake, which with some jet drives can't be performed while aboard—you'll have to get wet to do it. Finally, handling at low speeds is a bit sloppy because of the weak water flow out of the nozzle.

But these are minor handicaps for some anglers, who love the ability to fly through shallows and corner around obstructions. Manufacturers are coming out with more outboard and stern-drive jets every year, and they're selling incredibly well.

THE PROPELLER

The propeller, also referred to as the screw or the wheel, is integral to optimal boat performance. The propeller should be matched to the boat, not necessarily the motor. As a matter of fact, some high-horsepower motors are sold without propellers so that the boat dealer or owner can choose the best propeller for the craft. A boat with an incorrect propeller may take a long time to reach plane, not attain cruising speed, create cavitation (see page 39), or otherwise not operate efficiently. The wrong prop could also cause internal damage to your engine.

According to propeller experts, owners of boats that are rated for motors of less than approximately 30 horsepower have no need to worry about poor prop performance; the propeller that comes with the outboard will work for most situations. Owners of larger craft should be sure that their propeller is correct for both their boat and their uses.

Propellers come in a variety of materials. The most common propellers today are made of *aluminum*, because they are inexpensive and efficient for their cost. Although aluminum props are somewhat soft and do not stand up well to impact, they are easy and inexpensive to repair.

Stainless steel propellers, because of their integral strength, stand up to abuse much better than do aluminum props. They also offer better performance, and many owners of bass boats and other craft for which speed and handling are priorities choose stainless steel. The "hole shot," which is the acceleration of a boat from standstill to planing mode, is accomplished quickly with a stainless-steel propeller (more on hole shots later).

So if your fishing involves traveling through obstruction-filled, prop-knocking waters, where damaging your propeller is a question of *when* instead of *if*, which propeller is better? Stainless props are tough and will shrug off many impacts, but they are not indestructible. And they are much more costly to repair than aluminum—though damaging an aluminum prop every time you head out will cost plenty, too. Unfortunately, there is no clearcut answer.

Relatively new on the scene are *composite* propellers, which offer the advantages of light weight and imperviousness to corrosion. They are relatively inexpensive, and many have impact

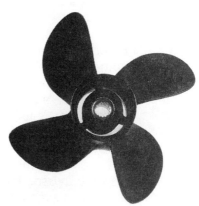

Most propellers today are either aluminum or stainless steel. Although stainless props generally offer better performance, modern technology has improved the aluminum prop. This Quad-R-Jet four-blade aluminum prop from Propco, said to be the first of its kind, is supposed to offer the performance of steel at the price of aluminum.

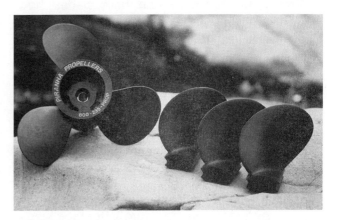

Composite propellers are lightweight and impervious to corrosion. This composite prop, the Piranha B14x11, offers the advantage of replaceable blades. If a blade is damaged, the owner replaces only that blade instead of fixing or replacing the entire prop.

resistance on a par with aluminum props. At least one manufacturer of composite propellers makes a model with blades that are individually replaceable. Fishermen can keep spare blades on board and replace damaged ones; replacement blades are fairly inexpensive.

Plastic propellers are used on electric trolling motors and occasionally as emergency replacements for metallic or composite props. If damaged, they cannot be repaired.

The number of blades on a propeller affects its performance. This number ranges from two to six. Basically, the fewer blades, the faster the speed attainable by the boat. Conversely, the more numerous the blades, the better the "bite" in the water, because there is more blade surface. This results in a smoother ride with better handling qualities. But more blades result in more prop "drag." For all-around, average use, the three-blade propeller provides the most reasonable compromise between efficient running and smooth riding.

Propellers with more than three blades, however, are becoming increasingly common, especially on high-performance craft such as bass boats. The reason is that these multibladed propellers provide an improved hole shot, because of their good bite in the water.

A number of terms define propeller configuration:

Propeller *diameter* is straightforward: the diameter of a circle made by the spinning propeller blades. The larger the diameter, the more surface area, which increases drag but assists in getting the boat moving. Boats heavy for their size need large-diameter props, while boats that are built for speed need small-diameter props for their size.

Pitch is the distance, measured in inches, that a propeller would move in one complete revolution *through a solid medium*. For example, a propeller with fifteen-inch pitch would theoretically travel fifteen inches through a solid medium in one turn. In water, however, the propeller would travel less than that distance. The difference between theoretical distance and actual distance is called *slip*. On most boats, slip varies between 10 and 30 percent. Heavy hulls slip less than quick-planing hulls. Slip is actually necessary to develop thrust.

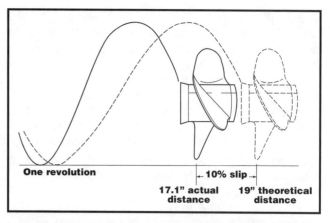

Propeller slip is the difference between the theoretical travel of a propeller (called pitch) and the actual travel of that propeller after one revolution.

Pitch and slip are important because the proper amount of each will provide best performance. A low pitch provides a good hole shot and acceleration; a high pitch will increase top speed, though it will take more time getting there. But there is potential for engine damage in either extreme. If the propeller is of too low a pitch for the boat, the engine has the potential to overwork. If the prop is of too high a pitch, the engine will lug down. Both situations will shorten the life of the engine.

Some propellers are *cupped*, which refers to a curl on the trailing edges of the blades. Cupping has the same effect as increasing prop pitch. It also allows the propeller to hold better in the water when it is not completely submerged, as cupping provides an improved bite.

Propeller *rake* is the angle, measured in degrees, of the propeller blades in relation to the hub. Propellers at a right angle to the hub have zero rake; propellers that angle back, or aft, have positive or progressive rake; and propellers that angle forward have negative rake. Positive rake is most common, and most general-performance propellers average about 15 degrees of rake. Positive rake allows a motor to be mounted higher on the transom because the angled-back blades lessen cavitation problems. High-performance craft such as bass boats usually have propellers with a higher degree of rake so as to allow improved planing abilities.

Propeller technology has improved tremendously over the years, yet has become increasingly complex as well. Propeller manufacturers and reputable boat dealers can assist your search for the best propeller for your boat.

Cavitation

Cavitation, or propeller ventilation, occurs when air from the water surface or exhaust gases from the motor are sucked or forced into the propeller area. This causes the propeller to lose full contact with water and thus decreases thrust. A common symptom of cavitation is an undue amount of water turbulence and noise at the propeller.

Cavitation is often easily remedied by adjusting the motor trim, or the angle of the motor in relation to the water surface. The antiventilation plate—the horizontally mounted steel plate above the propeller—on outboards and stern drives serves to reduce the induction of air to the propeller.

5

TRAILERS AND TOWING

As one of our definitions of a freshwater fishing boat is that the craft must be trailerable, the boat trailer and the hitch that connects it to the towing vehicle are important segments of the fishing boat package. Obviously a trailer is necessary to bring the boat to water, launch the boat, load it, and bring it back home again. But just as important is the fact that for the majority of boat-owning fishermen, the trailer is where the boat will spend most of its time.

In some respects, choosing the proper trailer for a boat is no longer a complicated or painful exercise. For instance, many boat manufacturers now sell boat packages, in which the boat, motor, and trailer are available for one price, and all the components are custom matched. The trailer is perfectly compatible with the craft. Boat dealers also assemble and sell boat/motor/trailer packages. In either case, the job of picking the right trailer has been done, and done right.

But many fishermen will buy a boat separately.

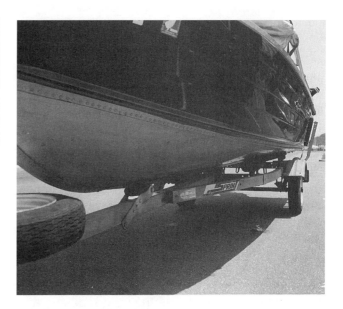

Your boat is, well, like a fish out of water when it rests on a trailer. The right trailer and hitch, as well as proper trailering techniques, are essential.

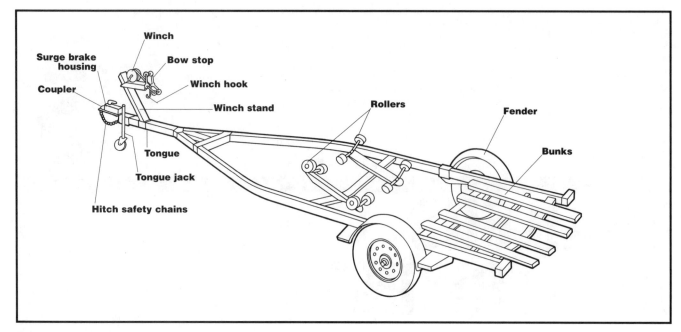

A trailer and its major components.

And we wouldn't see broken-down trailers at roadsides, or mishaps at launch ramps, if trailer matching and using was a no-brainer. Knowing a little bit about trailers and hitches will pay off in safe and uneventful traveling, launching, and loading.

TRAILER TYPES

Almost all manufactured boat trailers are made from steel channel stock, either painted or galvanized. Freshwater boaters don't need the protection of galvanized steel, as long as they don't ever launch in highly corrosive salt or brackish waters.

The bunk trailer is the simplest and most common trailer used for boats. It is used for relatively lightweight boats, as the boat slides up and rests on carpeted bunks. The bunks themselves can be adjusted to the best position for support-

ing the hull and properly balancing the boat on the trailer.

Because the bunk trailer must be submerged enough when launching to enable the boat to float off the bunks, the bunk trailer is not compatible with large, heavy boats or with shallow launching situations.

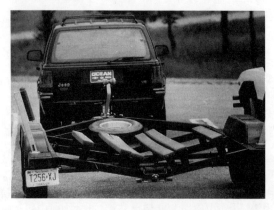

A bunk trailer is used for lightweight boats.

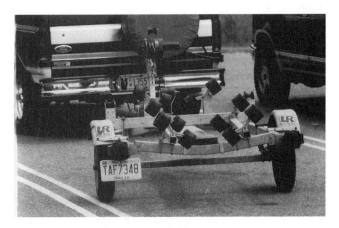

The roller trailer supports heavy boats and is ideal for launching in shallow water.

The roller trailer supports the boat with sets of rollers instead of bunks. Roller trailers are ideal for use with heavy boats, as the craft can be pushed right off the trailer and into the water. For the same reason, roller trailers are perfect for use in shallow-water launches. They also lessen the need for the boat launcher to wade around the launch site to shove the boat off the trailer.

Flatbed trailers, though commonly used for small one-person craft such as Jet Skis, aren't suitable for fishing boats because their design won't provide adequate support.

Many bunk and roller trailers designed for fishing boats have at least one *keel roller*, which as its name implies guides the boat's keel and thus the entire boat on and off the trailer. The heavier the boat, the more keel rollers necessary. Some trailers are hinged at about the midpoint of their length and can tilt down as the boat is being launched, which allows easy launching in shallow areas.

Whatever the type, most trailers carry a certification label showing their weight capacity. The trailer should be capable of carrying the boat plus all gear that you intend to place in the craft when you trailer it—motor, fuel, batteries, fishing gear, etc. However, playing it too safe and getting a trailer with a much higher capacity than the boat will result in a harsh ride and unnecessarily poor performance of the towing vehicle.

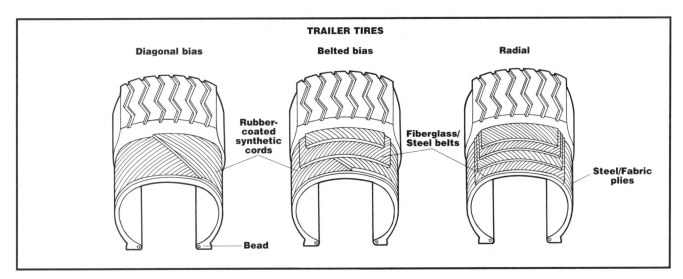

TRAILER TIRES

Diagonal bias — Belted bias — Radial

Rubber-coated synthetic cords

Fiberglass/Steel belts

Steel/Fabric plies

Bead

A trailer has comparatively small tires, which means they revolve more than the tow vehicle's tires. Investment in quality radials is advisable.

TRAILER COMPONENTS

Good *tires* are integral to safe and practical trailering. Most trailers wear tires that are smaller than automobile tires, because smaller tires keep the center of gravity lower on the trailer. A high trailer can cause a number of problems when towing, such as instability when making turns and when encountering crosswinds, and makes launching the boat in shallow water that much more difficult.

Smaller trailer tires must revolve more than the vehicle's tires, which subjects them to more wear. Though most trailer tires are well made, the driver must keep a close eye on their condition. Driving long distances on hot summer days can weaken a tire's construction. Be sure to follow the manufacturer's directions regarding inflation and tire rotation recommendations.

The wheel *bearings* can also suffer harm if no precautions are taken, especially if the wheels are routinely submerged when launching. Bearings should be checked and repacked with quality bearing grease at least every year and inspected for undue heat during long trips. Bearing protectors, commonly known by the brand name Bearing Buddy, are devices that fit over the hub and eliminate the need to frequently repack the bearings with grease. They also help keep water and dirt out of the bearings. Grease fittings allow for easy insertion of grease and quick checking of lubricant level, and have a relief valve to prevent overfilling. These bearing protectors are a smart investment and definitely worth their low cost.

A trailer that has a Gross Vehicle Weight Rating (GVWR, which is the sum of the trailer's weight plus its maximum carrying capacity) of 1,500 pounds or more is usually equipped with its own *braking system*. Most boat trailers have hydraulic surge brakes, which are activated by inertia: when the tow vehicle's brakes are applied, inertia causes a plunger-type device on the trailer to

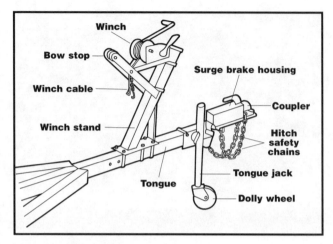

A typical trailer tongue and its components.

move forward and engage the brakes. Some heavy-load trailers have electric brakes, which are activated by pushing a button on the floor of the tow vehicle or are synchronized to the tow vehicle's brakes. A control allows the driver to adjust the trailer braking from soft to aggressive, depending on the load and the driver's needs.

Most trailer *suspensions* are of the leaf-spring variety. The axle rests on one or more spring-steel leaves, which are connected to the trailer frame. The leaves flex when the wheel hits a bump. The larger the trailer, the more leaves necessary. One advantage of leaf-spring suspensions on trailers is that no shock absorbers are necessary, as the friction between the leaves (which are shorter and stiffer than those found on automobiles) reduces sway and bounce.

Some large trailers employ coil-spring suspensions. These are lighter than leaf-spring suspensions and work well, but shock absorbers are necessary because there is no friction to reduce sway. Other hardware is necessary to hold the axle in the correct position. The complexities of a coil-spring suspension, plus its vulnerabiliy to damage from water immersion, make a leaf-spring setup a better choice in most situations.

Torsion-bar suspensions are found on a few new boat trailers. They are effective, quiet, and maintenance-free. Road shock is absorbed via an exterior axle that encloses a steel shaft surrounded by rubber. Basically, when the wheel hits a bump, the steel shaft twists, and the rubber absorbs the force.

All trailers must be equipped with a *lighting system*, which is connected to the tow vehicle's lighting wires. The minimum needs are running lights, stop (brake) lights, and turn signals. A four-prong plug connects the trailer's lighting system to that of the tow vehicle. Some trailers that have more lights have five- or seven-pronged plugs. Adapter kits allow easy connection to the tow vehicle, or the trailer dealer will install the system for a fee. Lights should be checked before and during trips, and especially after the trailer has been submerged, as seals could fail and shorts may occur.

On the tongue, or forward part of the trailer, is the trailer *winch*. This spool of rope, wire cable, or length of strap is necessary to pull the boat onto the trailer when loading. Some winches are hand-operated with a crank; others have an electric motor that winds in the cable. Owners of small boats will have no strain winding in their craft with a manual winch, while larger boats are more easily loaded with an electric.

Winches come in a variety of sizes and gear ratios. For lightweight boats—say, five hundred pounds—a 2:1 ratio (the winch drum turns once for every two turns of the crank) works fine. Boats weighing one thousand pounds and more will require a gear ratio of 4:1 or more. This makes the crank easier to turn, but requires more turns of the crank to load the boat. Some winches are two-speed (actually two gear ratios), so that the boat operator can use the lower gear to pull the boat up onto the bunks or rollers, then switch to a higher gear to move the boat forward.

Winch lines vary as well; each has its pros and cons. Wire cable is strong and won't rot from sunlight or chemicals, but its narrow diameter makes it hard to hold when guiding a boat onto a trailer. It also can abrade, with broken pieces of wire strands ready to impale your palm and fingers. On the other (unbloodied) hand, synthetic rope is easier to grasp and kinder to the skin, but can abrade and rot. Nylon straps are strong and durable, but they must be kept straight when cranking onto the winch drum—not always an easy task.

The winch itself is attached to the trailer on a *winch stand*. A *bow stop*, which meets the front end of the boat when it is totally on the trailer, is mounted on the winch stand.

A *trailer tongue jack* allows the trailer to be kept upright and mobile when not attached to the tow vehicle. Consisting of a basic jack apparatus with a wheel at the base, the tongue jack is mounted on the end of the tongue, just before the coupler. The jack is raised and lowered by turning a hand crank. A tongue jack makes connecting and disconnecting a trailer to the tow vehicle a simple, even a one-person, job. The operator simply jacks the tongue up to a level just over the hitch ball on the tow vehicle, moves the tongue over the ball, then drops it down.

At the very tip of the trailer tongue is the *coupler*, a concave device that fits over the hitch ball on the tow vehicle. It is the primary contact point between vehicle and trailer. Most couplers are of the lever variety, which attach to the hitch ball via a lever-and-spring system. A separate safety latch, when engaged, holds the lever in the down position.

Lever couplers provide for easy and quick mounting and dismounting of the trailer. Additionally, lever couplers allow a padlock to be placed through the latch, a recommended security measure when you must temporarily leave the trailered boat unguarded.

THE HITCH

Hitches are devices that are permanently attached to the tow vehicle and allow the connection of a trailer. There are four classes of hitches, each of which permits a certain weight to be towed, and several types of hitch devices themselves.

Before delving into hitches and figuring out which class and type are best for you, you should understand the weight ratings used to define hitch capacity. *Trailer weight* is the weight of the trailer and its load: boat, motor, gear. *Tongue weight* refers to the weight placed by the loaded trailer, via the tongue, onto the hitch ball.

Generally, tongue weight should be about 10 percent of the trailer weight. The reason for this rate is that too little tongue weight may cause the trailer to sway when being towed. On the other hand, too much tongue weight may cause the front of the tow vehicle to rise, which will reduce steering control. Fortunately, most boat trailers come properly balanced for an empty boat, so if your trailer matches your craft this shouldn't be a consideration.

HITCH CLASSES AND TYPES

A Class I hitch is sufficient to tow up to 2,000 pounds; Class II, up to 3,500 pounds; Class III, 5,000 pounds; Class IV, 10,000 pounds. Most freshwater fishing boats can be towed with Class II and Class III hitches.

Class I hitches are usually attached solely to

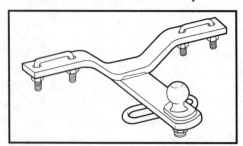

A Class I hitch is sufficient for towing up to 2,000 pounds.

the bumper of the vehicle, although some are also connected to the vehicle's frame. A hitch ball mounted on a step bumper (of the type found on many pickup trucks and sport/utility vehicles) usually falls into the Class I division and offers more strength than a regular bumper-mount hitch. Small utility boats, johnboats, canoes, and other craft of this size can be towed with a Class I hitch.

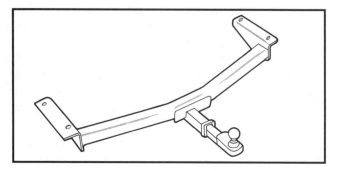

The Class II hitch can handle up to 3,500 pounds.

Class II hitches are attached to both bumper and frame or to frame only. Some sturdy step bumpers fall into the Class II division. Large utility boats and johnboats, multispecies boats and some bass boats are candidates for a Class II hitch.

The Class III hitch is attached solely to the frame. In this hitch class are two variations: the fixed-ball hitch and the receiver hitch. The fixed-ball type is simply a hitch ball bolted on to the hitch platform. The receiver hitch has a removable hitch-ball platform or bar that slides into the receiver.

There are some worthy advantages to the receiver hitch. First, the hitch ball and bar can be easily removed from the vehicle when towing is not required, which will prevent the formation of rust on the hitch ball. It will also prevent the bruising and bloodying of your shins when reaching into your trunk or rear storage area, as hitch-ball

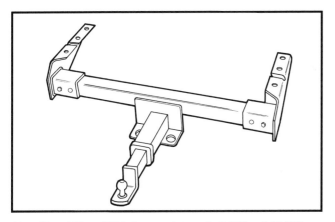

Class III and Class IV hitches can tow up to 5,000 and 10,000 pounds respectively.

mounts protruding from the rear of a vehicle have many hard and sharp edges. And employing a different size hitch ball is quickly accomplished—you simply slide one hitch bar out and pop another one in.

As Class III hitches can tow up to 5,000 pounds, they are appropriate for all but the largest of boats.

Class IV hitches also attach to the frame and are the strongest of hitches. Here (and with some Class III hitches as well) the hitch may be of the weight-distributing variety, which distributes tongue weight farther forward on the vehicle's chassis via spring bars.

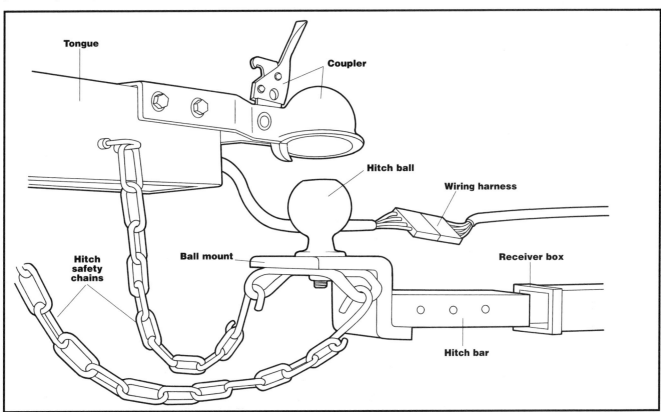

The trailer and the tow vehicle make all connections at the hitch.

HITCH BALLS

The hitch ball, stainless steel with a threaded neck, is bolted on to either the hitch itself or the hitch bar on receiver hitches. The two most common sizes are $1^7/_8$-inch and 2-inch diameters. Obviously the size of the hitch ball should match the hitch coupler. Neck sizes vary as well; generally the wider the neck, the stronger the ball.

SAFETY CHAINS

Chains should always be used as a precaution in the

event that the trailer disconnects from the tow vehicle while under way. The breaking strength of the chain should exceed the total weight of the trailer.

Two lengths of chain should be used. Each should be attached to the vehicle at a point on the frame, not the bumper, and to the trailer at the tongue. The chains should cross each other and create a cradle under the tongue. This will hold the tongue off the ground in the event of a mishap.

TOWING BASICS

You have your boat on your trailer, hooked up to

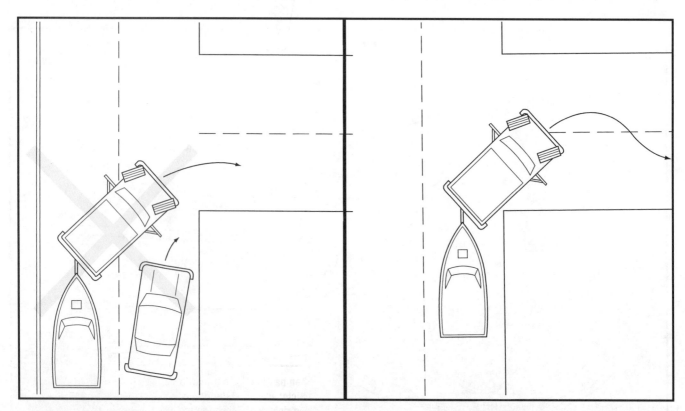

Your trailer will go everywhere your vehicle does and some places it doesn't, so you should allow extra room when turning. However, do not make a right-hand turn from a left-hand lane. Instead, stay in the right lane with your turn signal on and pause if necessary for any oncoming traffic in the road you are turning in to. When your way is clear, swing wide into the opposite lane to complete the turn.

your vehicle, ready to go find some water and fish. You jump in behind the wheel and go. A few minutes later you make a sharp turn and hear a *bang* as the trailer's wheels jump the curb.

It has happened to many of us, so don't be embarrassed (but do stop and check the trailer's tires and make sure the boat hasn't shifted). Towing a boat on a trailer isn't all that difficult, and following a few rules will ensure that nothing more than your pride will get hurt, if that.

1. Slow down. Carrying all that weight will alter the handling characteristics of your vehicle—acceleration, steering, and stopping—which means that you need more time to adjust to these changes. The only way to gain more time is to decrease your speed accordingly. You don't have to crawl along like a tortoise, but neither should you go as fast as you would without the trailer. Excessive speed is foolhardy when trailering, as the trailer may begin a swaying motion that will be impossible to control.

2. Give yourself space. The trailer will go everywhere your vehicle does and some places it doesn't. Because trailers will take a narrower turn radius than will your vehicle, you should swing turns wide. However, do not swing so wide that you will make a right-hand turn from a left-hand lane, as any vehicle trying to pass you on the right—and don't think this will never happen—will be hit by your trailer. (Never trust other drivers to see and honor your turn signal; it may be burned out anyway.) Instead, swing wide into the far lane of the road you are turning in to. If there is oncoming traffic, wait for it to clear.

   Also, give yourself space on the highway for entering, exiting, and changing lanes, as the length of your vehicle and trailer combined may be twice the length of what you are used to controlling. Check your mirrors care-

fully and signal your turn in advance, but not so much in advance that other drivers will think you inadvertently left the signal on from a turn half an hour ago.

3. Brake gently but firmly. Besides your needing the extra space to stop, you don't want to stand on the brake pedal when you have to stop suddenly. Conversely, you don't want to be tapping the brake pedal constantly. Brake gradually and with steadily increasing pres-

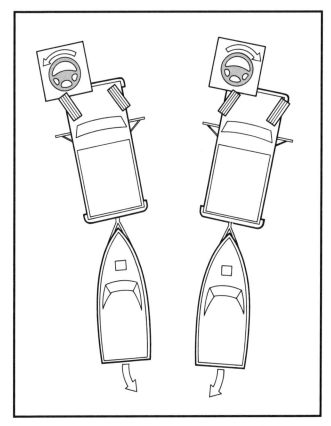

When backing up, a trailer turns exactly opposite from the tow vehicle: when the steering wheel is turned to the left, the trailer goes right; when the steering wheel is turned to the right, the trailer goes left. One trick: steering with your hand at the bottom of the steering wheel means that the trailer will go in the same direction that your hand moves.

sure, pumping if necessary, until you come to a smooth stop. This also allows the trailer brakes to engage normally and in cadence with the vehicle brakes.

BACKING UP

Backing a trailer down a launch ramp or into a parking spot is easy in theory but can be difficult in practice. The reason is that in reverse, the trailer responds to the turn of the towing vehicle's steering wheel by turning in the opposite direction from the vehicle (see diagram). The best method, which you should practice in a large empty parking lot, is to put your hand on the bottom of the steering wheel. In this manner the trailer will move in the direction that you move your hand when backing up: when your hand moves left, the trailer moves left; move it right and the trailer moves right.

Narrow boat launches, with limited space for maneuvering the trailered boat for a straight shot down the ramp, can prove challenging at best, especially when other fishermen are waiting for their turn. One tip here: if possible, back the boat down to the ramp from the left (driver's) side so you can look out the side window and make minor corrections when necessary. But even this is not simple if you're not familiar with the technique, so it bears repeating: invest some time practicing the maneuvers in an empty parking lot.

An excellent source of detailed information on trailers, hitches, and towing is the *Trailerboat Guide* by Joe Skorupa, part of the Hearst Marine Books series. It is available where you bought this book, or you can contact the publisher: Hearst Marine Books, 1350 Avenue of the Americas, New York, N.Y. 10019.

6

FISHING BOAT OPTIONS AND ACCESSORIES

Outfitting your boat with the proper fishing equipment can seem like an enjoyable task, but may prove perplexing after you've pored over marine catalogs or strolled through a boating equipment store. Fortunately, many new fishing boats now come equipped (or can be ordered) with major fishing accessories, such as livewells and boat seats. But it's the small stuff, which you either truly need or suddenly realize that you can't live (or fish) without, that can tear a huge chunk out of your budget if you don't shop and choose carefully. Remember that there are very few bargains in marine equipment: investing in a quality item will most often save you more money, over the long term, than will buying an attractively priced piece of gear on impulse.

ROD HOLDERS

Rod holders serve several purposes: they hold fishing rods in safe and out-of-the-way areas, keeping the rods from bouncing around in the bottom of the boat; they hold prerigged rods at the ready so a fisherman can pull a rod from its holder and begin fishing immediately; and they hold rods securely when actively fishing, such as when drifting or trolling. This last purpose also allows the boater to fish several rods at once without having to hold a fishing rod in his hand while tending to other duties, such as steering the boat.

Basically there are three types of rod holders. No one design is better than the others; each type satisfies different needs of fishermen and suits a certain style of boat.

The clamp-on rod holder, for example, is designed to quickly and easily mount anywhere on a boat's gunwale via a C-type clamp. Usually a wing nut that holds the rod bracket to the C-clamp allows a great amount of horizontal and vertical adjustment of the rod angle; you simply

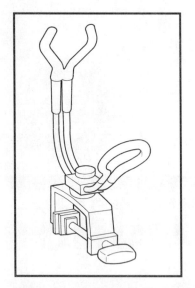

The clamp-on rod holder mounts anywhere on a boat's gunwale.

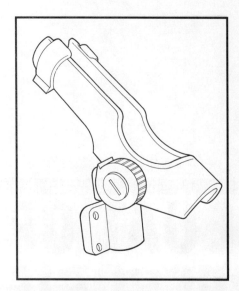

The two-piece rod holder is mounted on a permanent base and is a bit more reliable than the clamp-on variety.

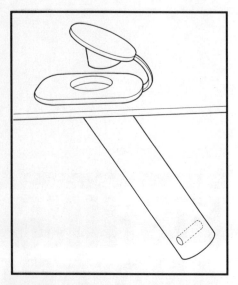

The flush-mount rod holder fits inside the gunwale and holds the rod securely at an angle.

loosen the wing nut, adjust the rod bracket, and tighten. Clamp-ons also can be removed as quickly as they can be installed. But there are some disadvantages to them: in rough water or when a large fish strikes, the rod can bounce out of the front fork, in which the rod shaft rests. Also, removing the rod butt from the rear O-ring on the bracket requires the fisherman to push the rod away before pulling it back. If you're drifting or trolling and a fish strikes on a rod in the holder, such a delay in setting the hook can result in a lost fish. Finally, most clamp-ons fit only on boats with narrow gunwales, such as johnboats and utility boats.

Two-piece rod holders are a bit more integral in that a base is permanently mounted somewhere on the boat gunwale, either on the top or on the side. The rod bracket locks into the base, usually via a post or by turning a locking wheel. The bracket is often a cylinder affair that is open along most of its length, allowing the fisherman to simply lay the rod in the holder. Many models have a ring at the top of the rod bracket that can be turned closed, which secures the rod in the bracket. Two-piece holders are usually more sturdy than clamp-on holders, and an angler can customize placement of the holders by installing a number of bases at key positions along the gunwale, both on top and on the side. Because of the base system, two-piece holders can be installed on practically any craft.

Flush-mount rod holders consist of a tube that fits in the gunwale itself. The top of the tube is flush with the top of the gunnel. A small rod sits crossways inside the tube, which the rod butt rests against to prevent the fishing reel body from making contact with the gunwale. The tube itself is usually angled toward the stern and out to the side of the boat, to facilitate trolling. Flush-mount holders are generally the most secure of all rod holders, as most of the length of the rod butt is firmly held inside the tube.

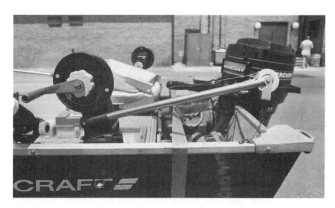

A downrigger close up. Mounted on a swivel base, the boom swings out perpendicular to the gunwale.

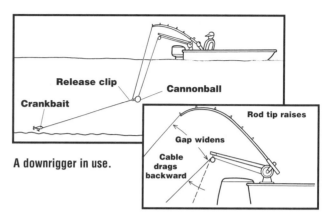

A downrigger in use.

A downrigger with a fish on it.

DOWNRIGGERS

A downrigger is a device that facilitates trolling by allowing an angler to present a bait or lure deep in the water without attaching unnecessary weight to the fishing line. It consists of a heavy weight (often called a *cannonball*) attached to the end of a cable. The cannonball can be raised and lowered by cranking in or letting out cable from a downrigger unit on a boat. To fish, the angler attaches the fishing line to a release clip that is in turn attached to the cable a short distance above the cannonball. The angler lowers the cannonball to the appropriate depth while paying out line from the fishing reel. When the angler begins trolling, the fishing line tightens enough to put a bend in the rod but not so much that the line will release from the clip. When a fish strikes the lure, the line pops from the release clip, the rod springs up, the fish is hooked and the angler picks up the rod to play the fish.

Dowriggers have experienced a tremendous growth in popularity in the past ten years because of the versatility they allow the boating angler. Before downriggers, the angler had to use heavy fishing line—sometimes with a lead core—and an array of sinkers or other weights to present his bait or lure at deep levels. Even then, when a fish was hooked, all the added weight took a lot of the sport out of playing a fish; often it was simply a matter of winching in the fish like a log on a chain. With a downrigger, however, even ultralight tackle can be used to present a tiny lure at the bottom of a deep lake without adding weight to the line.

The downrigger unit itself consists of a large spool that holds the cable. Some spools are cranked by hand to raise the cannonball, though others turn via an electric motor. A rod holder on the downrigger unit keeps the rod in place when trolling. A long arm, or boom, projects out from the spool housing to keep the cable away from the boat. Most downriggers are mounted on the gunwale, via a base-plate system: the base is permanently mounted at an appropriate place on the gunwale, where the downrigger unit itself can be quickly attached or removed when it is not in use. Many anglers will mount two downriggers on their boat, one on either side of the stern. By mounting rod holders that angle out from the starboard and port sides of the boat, the angler can then troll with four fishing rods and four different baits or lures at various depths.

FISH LOCATORS

These electronic sonar units have probably affected modern fishing tactics and techniques more than any other device. Simply, a fish locator is a sonar device that allows the angler to view, on a video or liquid-crystal display screen, representations of objects in the water underneath the boat: the lake bottom, its structure, and fish. These units also give numerical readouts of the depth of the water in that location. The screen is constantly updated with new readings on a right-to-left scroll so that the angler can constantly keep track of the area he or she is in.

Fish locator technology has advanced quite rapidly over the last decade. The latest models operate like computers, with high-resolution color screens and viewing options shown on scroll-down menus. Many models offer features such as fish "alarms" and the ability to provide a view into the water both beneath the boat and to the

side of it. Some actually show a three-dimensional representation of the lake bottom, including fish throughout the water column.

Fish locators (also called depth finders, depth sounders, and fish finders) work by sending out sonar pulses and receiving their echoes, rendering them onto a screen in a display that fishermen can read. The sonar pulses themselves are transmitted through a transducer, which is wired to the fish locator and mounted on the side or the bottom of the boat. The fish-finder unit itself comes with a base that should be permanently mounted on the boat, preferably in a location that allows the angler to easily view the screen both when motoring and fishing. The unit can be quickly attached to the base and wired to the battery via leads just before fishing, and removed afterward. Owners of small craft such as johnboats, which don't offer many practical locations for a base to be mounted, can buy a portable unit that clamps on to a seat or gunwale.

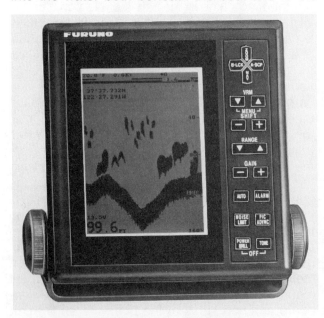

A fish finder, such as this Model LS-6000 from Furino, shows bottom structure as well as fish.

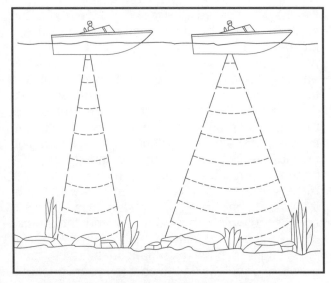

The transducer on a fish finder emits sonar pulses in a cone shape. This area is what the fisherman views on the unit's screen. Transducers with various cone angles are available. Narrower cones show less of the bottom but provide more detail.

Fish finders have become quite sophisticated. Learning how to use one properly is more time-consuming than it is difficult, so plan on spending some time with the instruction booklet. Keen competition among manufacturers has resulted in affordable prices for fish locators: an outlay of two hundred dollars will get you a unit with more features than you probably need right away. It's a worthwhile—practically necessary—investment for any boat angler.

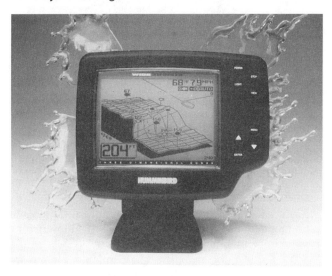

Some sonar units display the bottom and any fish in the area in "three-dimensional viewing." This is the Humminbird Wide 3D Vista model.

ANCHORS

While not necessarily a fishing-specific item, an anchor is an essential item on any fishing boat. An anchor, of course, allows the boat to remain stationary (or practically stationary) so a fisherman can cast to a specific section of water. But there's more to anchoring than just throwing one overboard and tying off, as a number of variables—wind, current, depth—can cause the

anchor to lose its hold. The next chapter deals with these anchoring techniques; here we will focus on anchor types themselves.

The mushroom anchor is probably the most common type used on freshwater boats. Resembling an inverted mushroom, it holds bottom solely by virtue of its weight and is most practical for use on sand and mud bottoms in little or no current, though it works fine on rocky bottoms in wind-free or current-free conditions. Most weigh ten to twenty pounds. The larger the boat, the larger the anchor needed to hold it—up to a point. Raising and lowering a fifty-pound anchor borders on the ridiculous, which is why other anchor designs become necessary with larger boats and/or in swifter currents.

The navy anchor has short and rounded opposing flukes attached to a rod that swivels at its base. This anchor holds a boat stationary because the heavy flukes will dig into a soft bottom as the boater pays out line while wind or

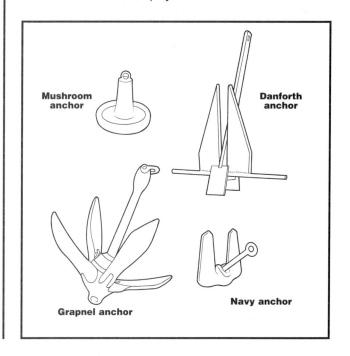

Mushroom anchor

Danforth anchor

Grapnel anchor

Navy anchor

current pushes the boat away. However, the navy anchor does not hold all that well in the lighter weights that are practical for small boats.

The Danforth anchor and its many variations are most popular for use with medium-sized and large fishing boats. Unlike the mushroom anchor (and the navy anchor to some extent), the Danforth does not utilize weight to hold a boat stationary. Instead the anchor's long, narrow, pointed flukes dig solidly into soft bottom once line is paid out, because the center rod will swivel with the movement. If wind or changing current move the boat while anchored, the Danforth will usually turn in the bottom and reposition itself. Danforth-type anchors also are comparatively lightweight and fold flat for easy storage.

A grapnel anchor is necessary to hold on rough or rocky bottoms or in rivers. This type works by virtue of three swiveling flukes that hook on to and hold bottom structure. Grapnel anchors also fold flat when stowed.

Navy, Danforth, and grapnel anchors all work better with a short length of chain attached to them, because the weight of the chain will force the anchor to tip on its side, which is necessary for it to dig into the bottom and hold.

Other anchor types exist, but these four are the most common. And millions of small-boat owners get by just fine with a homemade anchor, often a concrete-filled coffee can with an eye bolt sunk into the top.

GPS

This new navigation system has a double benefit for fishermen: GPS (which stands for Global Positioning System) not only allows boaters to figure exact position on the water via latitude and longitude, but it also lets anglers record a particular spot on the water so they can return to it later. Moreover, it provides an easy method for boaters to return to shore through otherwise featureless water.

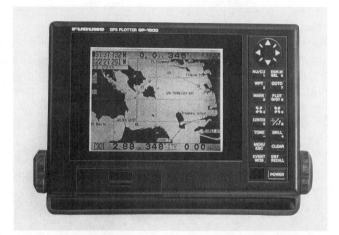

The GP-1800 Gps/plotter from Furino is one example of a GPS unit designed specifically for fishermen. When used with the proper digitized "chart cards," this unit will present a continuous display of the boat's position, speed, intended course, and past track, as well as representations of coastlines and depth contours.

A GPS unit works via high-frequency signals emanating from a number of orbiting military satellites. By triangulation and by figuring the time it takes for the signals to reach the GPS unit, it will compute latitude and longitude. (GPS is the technology used by the U.S. military to guide "smart bombs.") Some units are so small they can fit in a shirt pocket. Others incorporate an LCD screen on which maps can be viewed and a course can be plotted. Though the signals for civilian use guarantee accuracy within one hundred yards, it usually is much better.

(Loran, which stands for long range navigation, is a navigation system that has been in use for years. A loran unit receives low-frequency signals from land-based towers; the time differences are converted to latitude and longitude via triangulation. Loran offers the same benefits as GPS, but is not always as accurate and does not work on all waters. At this time the U.S. Coast Guard, which is the operating body for loran, is considering shutting down the loran system because of expense and the fact that GPS duplicates it. Any new boater who is in the market for a navigation system should invest in GPS instead of loran.)

GPS, with all its details and intricacies, deserves a book unto itself. Suffice it to say that a GPS unit is a worthwhile investment for the fisherman who plans to go out on big water.

TROLLING MOTORS

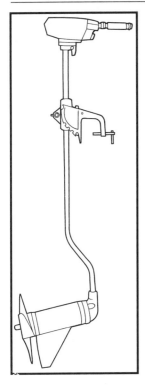

The electric trolling motor is more than a device to troll with. It also serves as an auxiliary motor to an outboard, the primary motor on a small boat, and a secondary motor when fishing small sections of large lakes. An angler can move short distances quickly and easily without starting up the primary motor, which could spook fish in some situations.

Trolling motors operate on a deep-cycle marine battery or a pair of them, depending on their strength. Most trolling motors are rated in terms of pounds of thrust instead of horsepower, which can make choosing the right one for your boat a bit difficult. One often-stated rule is that an electric troller should provide at least one pound of thrust per one hundred pounds of total boat weight, gear and anglers included. Thus a three-hundred-pound total weight requires a minimum thirty-pound-thrust electric.

Electric motors are lightweight and quiet running. This Evinrude model mounts on the transom.

Some of the largest electrics provide about sixty pounds of thrust, so obviously electric trolling motors are limited to use on smaller fishing boats.

There are many advantages to trolling motors. A flick of the switch turns them on, a simple tiller-mounted throttle allows easy maneuvering, and their electric operation guarantees quiet propulsion. Anglers who don't wish to invest in a gas-operated outboard can get by just fine on small waters with an electric. Electrics are lightweight, with most weighing less than thirty pounds (without battery). And because gas outboards are off limits on many waters these days, an electric can save you a lot of rowing. Maintenance is minimal; recharging the battery (via a battery charger that runs off household current or an automobile alternator) is the most tedious part of ownership. Still, a charged battery will keep a trolling motor operating at full capacity for at least a day of fishing, and with careful operation will push a boat for an entire weekend without pooping out.

Trolling was the primary purpose of these motors, but anglers have found them to be quite useful for other purposes. For instance: you want to work an entire shoreline for bass, casting to all

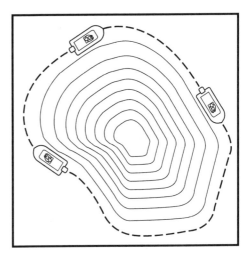

Some new trolling motors incorporate sonar systems, which can be programmed to follow a creek channel, cruise a shoreline, or circle a submerged hump, as shown here.

likely spots. A slight offshore wind constantly blows your boat away from your target, but anchoring in one spot limits you to one area. With an electric, you can keep your position in the wind and slowly move up or down the shoreline simply by turning the motor and giving it a bit more power. What's more, many electric trollers can be throttled and steered by an optional remote foot pedal, which means you don't have to stop casting to make the move.

Innovative electric motors on the market today incorporate electronic navigation systems. Some have a built-in electronic compass that will keep the motor on course in whichever direction you choose. Others have an internal sonar system that, when in use, can keep a boat over a specific water level, along a channel edge, or at the same distance from a particular shoreline. No additional manipulation of the motor is necessary.

LIVEWELLS AND BAITWELLS

As mentioned in Chapter 2, a number of new fishing boats come equipped with bait tanks and wells in which to keep the fish you catch.

Minnows and other live bait won't last long kept in a bucket; the angler must constantly change the water to keep the bait not just alive, but also in lively, fish-attracting condition. Also, many anglers like to keep their catches alive as long as possible. Tournament bass fishermen especially need a device to keep their fish alive, as catch-and-release is the rule of most bass tournaments nowadays. (The bass are released into the water after weigh-in.) But many anglers buy or own boats that don't come with livewells or baitwells. Fortunately, a number of aftermarket products exist.

Most portable baitwells are oval in shape, which protects the bait from striking walls and corners when the boat is in motion. Most come with an electronic aeration system to keep the water highly oxygenated, and are insulated to keep the water cool on warm days. Portable livewells can be fashioned out of an ice chest or similar large container and outfitted with a separate aeration system. Some manufacturers sell a kit that contains both a pump, to fill the container with water, and an aerator, to provide oxygen. All the angler needs is the container itself.

Mail-Order Companies

American Marine Electronics & Supply, Inc.
5700 Oleander Dr.
Wilmington, NC 28403
1-800/243-0264

Bass Pro Shops (Marine Catalog)
1935 S. Campbell
Springfield, MO 65898
1-800/227-7776

Cabela's (Marine and Fishing Catalog)
812-13 Ave.
Sidney, NE 69160
1-800/237-4444

Offshore Angler
1935 S. Campbell
Springfield, MO 65898
1-800/633-9131

Outer Banks Outfitters
Atlantic Station, P.O. Box 3330
Atlantic Beach, NC 28512
1-800/682-2225

Overton's
111 Red Banks Rd., P.O. Box 8228
Greenville, NC 27835
1-800/334-6541

West Marine
P.O. Box 50050
Watsonville, CA 95077
1-800/538-0775

7

BOAT-HANDLING SKILLS FOR ANGLERS

A fully equipped boat won't help you catch fish unless you are familiar with the methods of boat control and placement. Here we will cover the fundamentals.

ANCHORING

Dropping an anchor in a likely area is the most basic of boat-fishing methods. There's nothing amateurish about it, either; anchoring near a weedbed or point and casting out live bait or working the area thoroughly with lures is often the only method that pays off. The trick is knowing how to set an anchor properly.

First, an anchor line should always be tied off at the bow of the boat. Even a barely noticeable wind will push the boat back and away from the anchor, which means the boat will be subject to oncoming waves, whether natural or man-made, approaching from the bow. Because the bow of a boat is designed to ride through and over waves, your anchor will hold and boat occupants will remain comfortable. Anchoring from the stern or the sides will provide a rough anchorage and

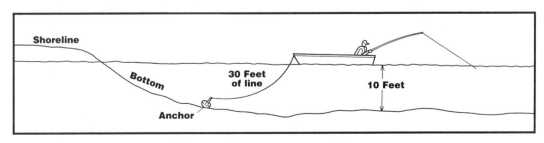

Setting an anchor in a pond or a quiet cove requires a scope—the ratio of water depth to anchor line—of only 3:1 to hold securely.

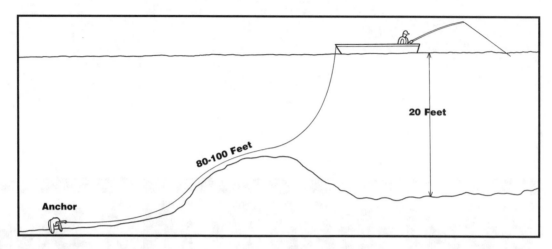

Holding bottom in the middle of a lake during windy conditions or heavy boat traffic may require a scope of as much as six or seven to one.

20 Feet

80-100 Feet

Anchor

possibly pop the anchor out at best, or cause the boat to swamp at worst.

The amount of anchor line you let out determines how well your anchor will set in the bottom. The ratio of anchor line ("rode" in nautical terms) to the depth of water (plus the distance from the bow to the water surface) is called *scope*. The correct ratio varies according to the size of boat, size and type of anchor, and the existence of wind or current. The minimum ratio is 3:1; that is,

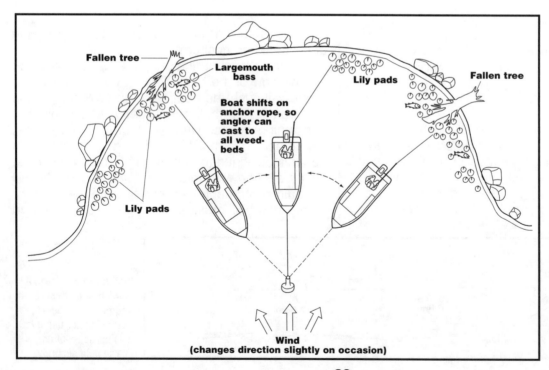

Fallen tree

Largemouth bass

Lily pads

Fallen tree

Boat shifts on anchor rope, so angler can cast to all weed-beds

Lily pads

Wind
(changes direction slightly on occasion)

Anglers can use the wind in their favor if the boat is positioned properly when anchored. Here, the boat will swing in an arc that allows the angler to cast to all likely fish-holding locations.

60

the amount of anchor line you let out should be three times the depth of the water you are anchoring in. For example, if you want to fish for largemouths in a quiet, weed-lined cove with a depth of about ten feet, you should let out thirty feet of anchor line to ensure a solid hold. If the wind picks up, you may have to release another ten feet of line, or the effect of the wind pushing on the boat may cause the anchor to lose its grip on the bottom. In extreme conditions—a large and heavy boat in the middle of a big lake, strong wind, choppy water from nearby boat traffic—you may need a scope of 7:1.

Even if an anchor is holding bottom properly, the boat will swing from side to side, again even in barely perceptible wind. This can be advantageous for fishermen, however, as the slow back-and-forth movement provides a wide area to fish.

As the boat swings in a prescribed arc, anglers can cast to the extreme edges of the range as well as the middle. This method works well when you suspect fish are in a general location but do not have them pinpointed. Let's say you're anchored in the middle of that weed-edged largemouth cove. It's an early morning in the summer and you suspect that the bass are prowling the edges of the lily pads. You have set the anchor and positioned the boat so that you can easily cast to the pad edges when the boat is in the middle of the arc, and you can reach other sections of the lily pads at either end of the arc with longer casts. Your plastic worm draws no hits as you cast it to the weeds and retrieve it along the bottom, but at the edge of an arc you can cast to a tree that has fallen into the water close to shore and—bang—a bass hits. Now you can narrow

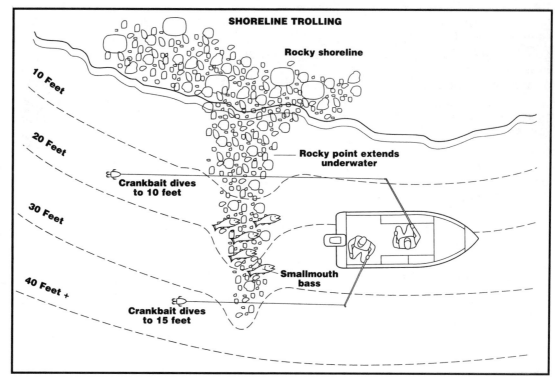

In this forward-trolling scenario the angler is fishing two rods to work a submerged point. By making repeated passes over points, increasing the distance from the shoreline with each pass, changing to deeper-diving lures when necessary, and experimenting with various trolling speeds, the angler should eventually get into fish—if they're in the mood to eat. Note that the lines are of different lengths to prevent tangling.

SHORELINE TROLLING

Rocky shoreline

10 Feet

20 Feet

Rocky point extends underwater

Crankbait dives to 10 feet

30 Feet

40 Feet +

Smallmouth bass

Crankbait dives to 15 feet

down likely areas to find largemouths that day: fallen trees and other wooden structures near weeds in what looks like five feet of water.

But there will be other times when you don't wish to allow the boat to swing from side to side, such as when fishing a small submerged rocky hump for walleyes. In this case you will need to drop a second anchor off the stern. If you are fishing relatively close to shore, you may tie off a second line on a solid shoreline object, go back out to your preferred fishing spot, and drop anchor there.

FORWARD TROLLING

The basic trolling technique is deceptively simple: you put a lure into the water, let out some fishing line, and row or motor slowly (with an outboard at low speed or with an electric trolling motor) through likely areas. When a fish grabs the lure, you stop rowing or put the engine in neutral and bring the fish in. Trolling is productive because you can cover a lot of potential fish-holding water in a short period of time, and the method allows you to pinpoint areas where fish are holding. Many anglers going after smallmouth bass, yellow perch, walleyes, lake trout, and other species will troll until they catch a fish, then anchor in that spot and cast.

But as with most methods, success lies in the details. First is the choice of trolling *lure*. A plastic worm, which is designed to be fished slowly on the bottom, is not a viable choice for trolling. The best lures for trolling are those that display an "action"— a side-to-side wobbling or a vertical diving—when in motion. Just as important is the *depth* of water you plan to troll. If you are fishing for walleyes that have located on structure in twenty feet of water, a crankbait that dives to a level of ten feet won't get even a look from the fish.

Trolling *speed* is another consideration. Generally, the faster the boat speed, the shallower the lures will run. This rule can be offset somewhat by using crankbaits that dive when retrieved or trolled, but there is a limit to their diving ability. (Many crankbaits of this nature come with directions that list their maximum running depth; check these before you buy.) Also, the longer line you troll with, the deeper the lure will run. Again, though, there is a maximum to this rule.

Forward-Trolling Techniques

Shoreline trolling is easily executed and generally productive. The angler simply steers the boat parallel to a shoreline, working into bays and coves and around points and shoreline obstructions. In this manner the trolled lures will run through practically the same depth of water, as long as the boat operator remains the same distance off the shoreline. Through trial and error, the trolling fisherman can eventually discover the depth at which fish are holding. For instance, let's say you plan to troll a large reservoir for smallmouth bass. You begin by setting out a pair of crankbaits, one that dives to five feet and another that dives to ten, and you troll in a pattern that keeps you twenty yards from shore. At this distance, the water is fifteen to twenty feet deep. If, after a reasonable amount of time, you don't catch a fish, begin a new trolling pattern thirty yards out from shore, where the water averages twenty to thirty feet deep. (You also change the five-foot-diving crankbait to one that dives to fifteen feet.) You round a rocky point, and the rod with the ten-foot-diving crankbait starts jumping (and as this is hypothetical, we'll call it a three-pound bass). Now you can assume that at least some smallmouths are holding about thirty yards off rocky points. You check with your depth finder (or with an anchor rope if you don't have electronics) and see that the water off the point where you hooked the bass is twenty feet deep. Now you can continue to troll, changing lures so that

Forward-Trolling Tips

1. Always begin trolling with at least two rods rigged with lures that dive to different depths. This allows you to cover two sections of the water column simultaneously.

2. Similarly, make sure the lines out from each rod are of different lengths, especially if you are trolling with lures that run at similar depths. Not only will this ensure that the lures cover different areas of the water column, it also will reduce the chance of the lines crossing one another and tangling when you make a turn.

3. Experiment with various trolling speeds. Just a minor increase or decrease in trolling speed will put your lures in different water columns and attract a strike.

4. Rod holders are handy places to insert rods when trolling—and necessary when trolling alone with more than one rod—but you'll increase your chance of solidly hooking a striking fish if you hold the rod in your hand. A slow trolling speed often does not impart enough energy to sink a hook past the barb. Holding the rod also allows you to impart additional action to the trolled lure, which may attract fish.

5. If you must keep your rods in rod holders when trolling, hit the throttle just a bit when a fish hits, then back down and grab the rod quickly. This increases the chances of a solid hookup.

both crankbaits dive to fifteen feet, and search out rocky points to troll. Or you can anchor off the point and cast similar crankbaits, or try jigs and/or live bait.

Zigzag (or S-curve) trolling is just what the name implies: steering the boat left and right in loose S-shape patterns until you find a fish. Zigzagging accomplishes two things: it allows you to cover a lot of water, so your lures will track through a lot of potential fish-holding areas; and the constant turning will allow your lures to range through various depths of the water column—they slow down and drop when you make a turn and speed up and rise when you straighten out. (Don't turn too tightly when zigzagging, or your lines will tangle.) When you do hook a fish, it's important to note the depth of the water and the speed of the boat (straight or turning) when the fish hit, as you should concentrate your further efforts at that depth and speed.

BACKTROLLING

Unlike forward trolling, in which the trolling lures follow the boat, backtrolling presents lures or bait to fish before the boat travels over them. In rivers, boaters backtroll into the current; in lakes, boaters backtroll into the wind. Lures are fished from the stern or the sides of the boat, and the slow backward movement allows the lures to range over and poke into most bottom contours and structure.

The technique is easily accomplished in rivers by facing the boat upstream, so the bow points into the current, and keeping the motor in forward gear (or rowing with oars into the current). The boater increases throttle until the craft maintains a neutral position, drops the lures into the water from the sides or stern, and then decreases a bit on the throttle. This allows the boat to slowly slip downstream at a much slower speed than that of

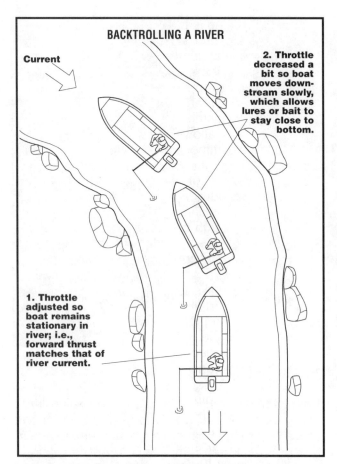

BACKTROLLING A RIVER

Current

2. Throttle decreased a bit so boat moves downstream slowly, which allows lures or bait to stay close to bottom.

1. Throttle adjusted so boat remains stationary in river; i.e., forward thrust matches that of river current.

When backtrolling in a river, the boat faces upstream with the motor in forward drive. Reducing the throttle until the boat moves slowly downstream allows the angler's lures or bait to remain close to bottom and be presented in all potential fish habitats.

the current. At any time the boat operator can increase throttle to hold steady, or turn the motor so that the lures can range from one side of the river to the other. Turning and pausing at the proper times and places allows the lures to range into all available fish habitat, even that close to shore.

Backtrolling in lakes against the wind takes more boat-handling skill, as wind is rarely as steady as river current. Also, wind changes direction frequently, creating sudden surges and slips of the boat. Because lakes have no current, the lures or bait must be fished below or just behind the boat. On lakes it is also possible, and sometimes much easier, to place the boat so the bow faces downwind and put the motor into reverse gear. In this manner the boater relies mainly on the motor instead of the wind for movement, but can still put lures or bait into all probable habitat.

DRIFTING

Fishing from a boat without benefit of anchor or power seems simple enough, but random floating is problematic: it's hazardous, as the craft moves to the whims of wind, waves, and swells from other passing boaters, which can put you into the path of an oncoming craft with no quick recourse for an evasive maneuver. Additionally, drifting at random probably will put you out of productive fishing areas more than it will get you in them. The solution, then, is a controlled drift over or near areas likely to harbor fish.

There are a number of ways to effect a controlled drift, but first keep in mind that boat *attitude*—the angle of the boat in relation to the drift—is vital to effective fishing, especially if more than one angler is in the boat. The craft should be presented broadside to the area being fished for advantageous and accurate casting.

Let's say a slight wind is steadily blowing parallel to the shoreline, and you wish to cast to the shallows near shore for largemouth bass. In this case, nothing more is necessary than to shut off the motor and begin casting. Because a boat will align itself to the wind (that is, the bow will eventually turn downwind), the port or starboard side of the boat will face the shoreline. Naturally, such perfect conditions rarely occur: the wind blows intermittently, or at an angle to the shoreline, or too hard for effective fishing, or not at all. Each of these problems can be overcome individually.

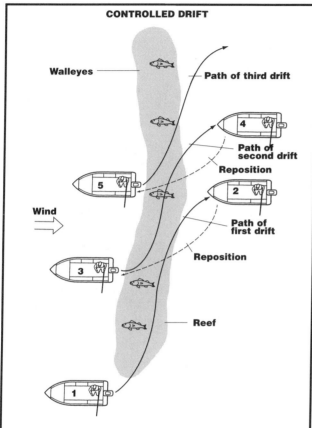

CONTROLLED DRIFT

Walleyes

Path of third drift

Path of second drift

Reposition

Path of first drift

Reposition

Wind

Reef

1. Boat is postioned at end of reef with electric motor turned at right angle to reef.
2. Combination of wind and motor thrust allows boat to drift over partial length of reef.
3. Boat repositioned near spot last fished.
4. Boat drifts over new section of reef.
5. Boat repositioned for final drift.

How to drift a submerged reef. Note that the repositioning paths cross that section of reef already drifted so as not to spook fish in the section not yet drifted.

First, if the wind is blowing intermittently or not at all, you can use an electric motor to make minor corrections to the drift or to move you along. Similarly, if the wind is blowing at an angle to the shoreline, you can use the electric to reposition yourself when the occasion arises. (A bow-mounted electric motor with a foot-operated remote control allows you to do this easily and without putting down your fishing rod.) Sometimes lifting the lower unit of the outboard out of the water, or keeping it turned to the extreme left or extreme right, will alter the course of the drift to your liking. So can keeping one oar in the water (though be careful not to lose it if it hits an obstruction).

If the wind is blowing too hard for an effective drift, you can use a *sea anchor* (also called a *drift sock*). These baglike devices are tied to the end of a line and open like a parachute when in the water, thus slowing the drift speed.

Another example: walleyes should be congregating on submerged islands or reefs offshore in a large reservoir, and you think they will respond to minnow-tipped jigs bounced across the bottom. With your depth finder on, you find one long but narrow hump that should hold fish, but high wind has created a chop on the water that makes it difficult to hold position—and the wind is blowing perpendicular to the reef. First, use your outboard to position the boat at the end of the reef, and shut it down so you don't spook the fish. Then face the boat into the wind and position your electric motor at almost a right angle to the stern, and increase or decrease power so that the boat eventually begins to move along the reef. You definitely will get blown off course eventually, but finding the right combination of electric motor power and boat angle to the wind should allow you to "drift" along at least some of the reef before the wind pushes you off. When it does, simply use the electric, or the outboard if necessary, to put the boat back into the spot last fished. This maneuver can be used over and over again until you have drifted over the entire reef.

Trimming Your Boat

Boat trim, or the angle of the boat in relation to the water, is crucial to a safe and comfortable ride as well as to good fuel economy. A boat at rest has a different angle on the water from a boat moving along on plane, so the motor should be adjusted so that the propeller shaft is parallel to the water's surface at cruising speed. At rest, the lower unit appears angled into the boat's hull.

High-horsepower outboards have "trim control," which allows the boat operator to adjust the angle of the outboard when under way. This is advantageous because larger boats have a wider weight-carrying capacity and experience a variety of water conditions, and the motor can be custom-trimmed to each situation.

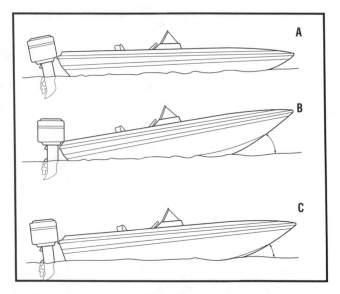

A. The bow is too low on this craft because the outboard motor is trimmed in too much. B. Here, the bow is too high because the motor is trimmed out too much. C. The outboard is trimmed properly.

8

PROFILES OF SELECTED FISH SPECIES

LARGEMOUTH BASS
(*Micropterus salmoides*)

The largemouth bass is the nation's number-one freshwater species as far as boating anglers are concerned. Native to warm-water lakes and rivers in the eastern and southern United States, the largemouth has a range that now extends to waters throughout the Lower 48 states, from half-acre farm ponds to miles-long reservoirs. Their preferred water temperature is 68 to 78 degrees F, though they will tolerate and actively feed in waters up to 80 degrees and down to the low to mid 60-degree range. Largemouths—which actually belong to the sunfish family, *Centrarchidae*—average one to three pounds, depending on the range, though larger fish are common in southern and western waters. The world record weighed twenty-two pounds four ounces and was caught in Montgomery Lake, Georgia, in 1932. Millions of

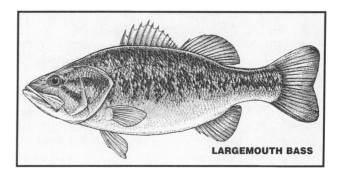

LARGEMOUTH BASS

anglers since then have tried to beat this record. A few have come close, with the largest bass coming from lakes in Florida and California.

Largemouths are not known for having a selective diet. Smaller fish, crustaceans, worms, insects, frogs, snakes, mice, and even small birds are all part of this gamefish's menu. However, many anglers have come home after a day of fishing with nothing to show for their efforts. Largemouths can "turn off" their feed, and nothing you throw at them will provoke a strike. Also, these fish change locations constantly. They will inhabit water from shallow to deep, depending on time of year, water type, and water temperature.

A largemouth angler's arsenal includes bait such as minnows, crayfish, frogs, and insects; and lures such as crankbaits, spoons, spinners, flies and plastic worms. This last bait is arguably the most effective largemouth bass lure throughout its range, usually fished on bottom with a slow retrieve.

SMALLMOUTH BASS (*Micropterus dolomieui*)

The smallmouth bass is indigenous only to the Lake Ontario and Ohio River drainages, though widespread stocking has introduced the "smallie" to waters from the Canadian border south to Alabama and Texas and west to California. The smallmouth prefers clean and cold water such as fast-moving rivers and spring-fed lakes with rocky bottoms. Preferred water temperatures are lower than that of the largemouth bass—65 to 73 degrees F—but you won't find smallmouths in lakes and rivers that heat up to much past 80 degrees, and in fact will catch them in water temperatures down to 55 degrees. A member of the sunfish family (as is the largemouth), the smallmouth gets its name from comparison to the largemouth: the "hinge" on the upper jaw extends past the eye on the largemouth, and falls even

with the eye on the smallmouth.

But that's the only small aspect of the smallmouth. One of the scrappiest fighters in freshwater, this bass will give a spirited battle all the way to the boat. A half-pound smallmouth—which is the average in many streams; about twice that in lakes—will give the fight of a largemouth two or three times its size. The world record smallmouth weighed eleven pounds fifteen ounces, and was caught in 1955 in Dale Hollow Lake, Kentucky.

Smallmouths prefer minnows, crayfish, worms, and assorted insects, with crayfish being the preferred forage where these crustaceans exist and when they are available. These baits, and lures resembling them such as jigs, spinners, and small crankbaits, all will take smallmouths.

WALLEYE (*Stizostedion vitreum*)

The walleye is the favorite gamefish of the northern Midwest states, though it has plenty of fans elsewhere in the country. Originally inhabiting the cool lakes and large rivers of the northern United States, the walleye has been introduced throughout the East and South and in parts of the West. This fish prefers clean, comparatively cool water—59 to 68 degrees F, though it will thrive in waters that reach the high 70-degree range—and must have access to deep water in order to spawn.

Often erroneously called the walleyed pike—it

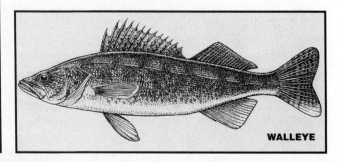

SMALLMOUTH BASS

WALLEYE

actually is a member of the perch family—the walleye gets its name from its oversized, moonlike eye. The species is favored table fare because of its mild and tasty white flesh. It also grows to decent sizes; these fish average two to three pounds in most areas. Larger specimens are taken frequently, though the ten-pound walleye is a benchmark trophy for most anglers. The largest walleye on record was caught in Old Hickory Lake, Tennessee, in 1960. It weighed a whopping twenty-five pounds.

Walleye are usually bottom oriented, feeding on minnows, worms, leeches, and the aquatic stages of insects. The angler would do well to use these baits, fished close to bottom. One of the most effective walleye offerings consists of a small jig "sweetened" with a minnow, nightcrawler, or leech, slowly bumped along the bottom. Small crankbaits and spinners, also fished close to bottom, will take walleyes as well. A slow presentation is the rule.

CHAIN PICKEREL
(*Esox niger*)

The chain pickerel is found throughout the eastern and southern states and is easily distinguished from its cousins in the pike family by the distinct chainlike markings on its flanks. With a long, wide mouth filled with long, sharp teeth, the pickerel averages around two pounds, with larger specimens reaching weights two and three times that. Pickerel like to ambush their prey and thus are denizens of the weedbeds, typically ponds, backwaters, and coves with depths ranging from two to fifteen feet or so. The chain pickerel is most active in water temperatures ranging from 66 to 80 degrees F, though they will thrive in waters well below those temperatures. The largest chain pickerel ever caught weighed nine pounds six ounces, taken in 1961 in Homerville, Georgia.

Surprisingly, few fishermen specifically pursue chain pickerel. These fish often are bycatches of anglers after largemouth bass, as the habitats of the two species overlap. One reason, perhaps, for the pickerel's relative unpopularity is that its flesh, while mild and tasty, is quite bony and difficult to prepare. Still, the pickerel provides plenty of sport and is a favorite of young anglers throughout its range because of its feeding habits, which are quick, ferocious, and frequent.

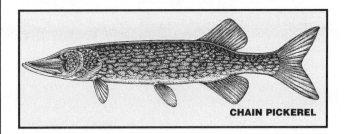

CHAIN PICKEREL

A favorite fishing method is also quite simple: hooking a shiner or other minnow a few feet below a bobber and casting it near or into a weedbed. In clear waters, and if the angler is attentive and quiet, it sometimes is possible to watch a pickerel "stalk" its prey and eventually pounce upon the minnow with lightning speed. Many other baits and lures will take pickerel, too. Diving crankbaits, spoons, and plastic worms are the most effective. Fly fishermen find great sport with pickerel as well by using large streamers fished slowly in and around the weeds.

NORTHERN PIKE
(*Esox lucius*)

Although they were originally found in the larger waters of the Northeast and northern Midwest states, stocking has broadened the range of the northern pike as far south as Pennsylvania and as far west as Montana, and Arizona. Like the

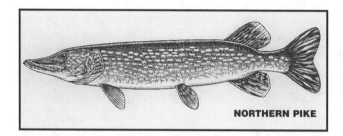

NORTHERN PIKE

chain pickerel, the northern pike has a long and thin body with a large, toothy mouth, but reaches much greater lengths and weights. It also shares the pickerel's voraciousness; the pike's tremendous appetite and attack style of feeding have earned it the nickname of "water wolf."

The average size of northern pike depends on the locale—two to four pounds in some waters, five to seven in others—though some lakes give up pike in the ten- to twenty-pound class routinely. The world record northern pike came from Sacandaga Reservoir in New York in 1940; it weighed forty-six pounds two ounces. Northerns range throughout the water column but seem to frequent weedbeds in lakes with close access to deep water, as well as humps or bars in deep river pools.

Northerns inhabit waters ranging from 50 to 70 degrees, and seem to prefer temperatures in the middle of that zone, from 55 to 65 degrees. These opportunistic predators do not have a finicky diet, except that they seem to prefer large forage (they have been known to eat ducklings). Yellow perch, suckers, and panfish are well known as favorite forage for northern pike. These fish, as well as large shiners and chubs, will take pike when fished with a bobber in the weeds or close to the bottom in pools and holes. Many fishermen prefer to use artificial lures for pike, with the red-and-white spoon being a time-honored favorite. Large spinners and crankbaits, especially those that resemble a yellow perch where that species is found, also take northern pike.

YELLOW PERCH
(*Perca flavescens*)

The yellow perch can be viewed as a transition species between gamefish and panfish in that it is pursued both for sport and for food. Found throughout the East and Midwest and in some western states, the yellow perch lives in all manner of lakes and ponds and in some rivers in its range. Schools of perch generally roam in search of food, often remaining in one area where forage is abundant, and the angler who lucks on to such a school can literally fill a bucket with them.

Perch prefer water temperatures from the mid-60- to the mid-70-degree range, with the midrange of this temperature zone the most favorable. Average weight for the species runs less than one pound, though a school of "jumbo" yellow perch may contain fish twice that weight. The world record yellow perch was caught way back in 1865 in Bordentown, New Jersey, and weighed four pounds three ounces.

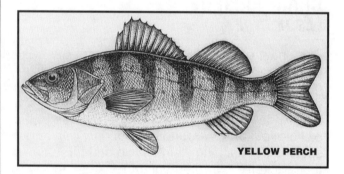

YELLOW PERCH

Yellow perch aren't very finicky feeders, but their forage is limited because of their comparatively small size. Small fish, insects, small crayfish, and snails make up a perch's diet. Probably the best bait for yellow perch is a small minnow fished live on a small hook, either suspended below a bobber or fished with weight close to the bottom. Small spinners, jigs plain or tipped with a minnow, and worms also take yellow perch.

Yellow perch are delicious, which is why many anglers strive to fill that bucket. Their firm, white flesh is considered one of the tastiest of all freshwater species. A commercial perch fishery exists on some northern waters, but is limited because of this species' comparatively diminutive size.

STRIPED BASS
(*Morone saxatilis*)

The striped bass is an anadromous species, meaning that it dwells in saltwater but ascends freshwater tributaries to spawn. Its original range is along the Eastern Seaboard and the southeast Gulf Coast, but the striped bass has been introduced to coastal waters on the West Coast and, most notably, in large freshwater lakes and reservoirs in the East and South. These "landlocked" stripers have thrived well beyond the expectation of fisheries managers and have created a large and popular fishery.

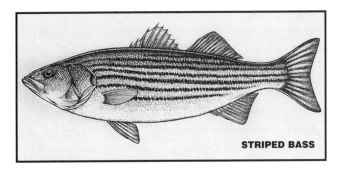

STRIPED BASS

In freshwater, striped bass don't get as large as their brothers in saltwater—at least in terms of record fish—but they do grow to tremendous sizes. Stripers range in weight from a couple of pounds up to the twenty-, thirty-, and forty-pound class and beyond. The world record freshwater striped bass was caught in 1988 in O'Neill Forebay, California, and weighed an even sixty-six pounds.

Freshwater striped bass are most active when water temperatures are in the 65- to 70-degree range, and a bit higher than that in warmer locales. The fish can be difficult to find, as they swim anywhere in the water column depending on temperature, time of year, and the forage present. This last can include any manner of fish, but is usually a specific species of baitfish such as gizzard shad that has been stocked along with the stripers to provide a large enough source of forage. Sometimes deep trolling with crankbaits and jigs is necessary to catch stripers; other times still-fishing with live or cut bait—large shiners, gizzard shad, even small trout where legal—can take them. At times a school of stripers will herd a school of baitfish to the surface, where anglers can catch them by casting surface or shallow-running lures at the commotion.

BLUEGILL
(*Lepomis macrochirus*)

Practically every state in the Lower 48 has waters that support a population of bluegills. This scrappy panfish is the most common species in farm ponds and smaller waters everywhere, and it is the rare fisherman who has not cut his angling teeth on bluegills. Hardy (they tolerate a wide range of water quality), abundant (one female bluegill may deposit as many as 38,000 eggs in her nest), very sporting for its size (it typically swims at right angles to the angler when hooked, and pulls extremely hard when doing so), and usually not finicky about feeding (insects, snails, small baitfish, worms, and, as many a kid has discovered, bread balls), bluegills provide about as much guaranteed sport as any species can. They also are superb table fare, ranking with the yellow perch and walleye in that category.

The downside, if any, is the bluegill's size. A one-pound bluegill is a whopper; unfortunately bluegills are so prolific that a population of them

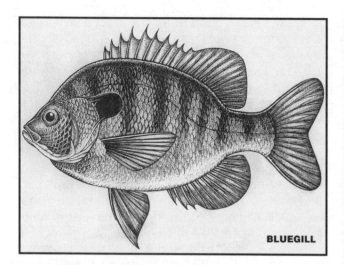

BLUEGILL

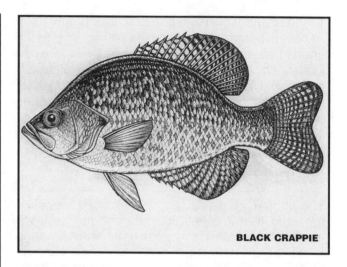

BLACK CRAPPIE

can quickly become stunted if fish are not removed regularly. The world record bluegill was caught in Ketona Lake, Alabama, in 1950, and weighed four pounds twelve ounces.

The angler going specifically after bluegills would be wise to check water temperatures. Although these fish are active in waters ranging from about 69 to 85 degrees F and even warmer, they are most comfortable in the 75- to 80-degree range. Best baits include garden worms and red worms, grasshoppers, crickets, grubs, and small minnows. Lure fishermen can use small jigs and spinners, miniature crankbaits, and small soft plastic baits. Fly fishermen can enjoy quick, tremendous sport by casting small dry flies, wet flies, and nymphs.

BLACK CRAPPIE
(*Pomoxis nigromaculatus*)

Also called the calico bass, the black crappie is a close cousin to the white crappie, and the two have been known to hybridize. Together the two panfish species provide millions of hours of early spring fishing (which is immediately prior to their spawning period) and in some waters constitute the primary target of fishermen. The reasons: crappies are not all that difficult to catch, once they are located; they are fun to fish for, as one school can provide hours of nonstop catching; and their flesh, while a bit on the soft side, is excellent.

Like most panfish, crappies do not grow to large sizes. A foot-long crappie, which is of admirable size anywhere, will weigh only a pound or so. The world record black crappie—which hasn't had a close competitor ever since it was taken—weighed six pounds even and was caught in Westwego Canal, Louisiana, in 1969. (The largest white crappie on record came from Enid Dam, Mississippi, in 1957, and weighed five pounds three ounces.)

Crappies range throughout the East, South, and Midwest states, and have been transplanted into a number of western waters. In spring these fish locate near cover prior to spawning: downed trees, weedbeds, undercut banks. Black and white crappies generally spawn when the water reaches the mid to upper 60-degree range. At other times look for black crappies in water temperatures from 70 to 75 degrees F; white crappies in 60- to 70-degree water.

Crappies forage on all manner of things—small fish, snails, small crayfish, and insects—but it's hard to beat a small live minnow, fished a few feet below a bobber, as a crappie bait. Some anglers troll very slowly with weighted minnows until catching a crappie, then they anchor and bobber-fish live minnows near the closest cover or bank. The best artificial lure for crappies is a small jig or a pair of them, fished with or without a bobber and slowly retrieved in the vicinity of shoreline or submerged cover.

BROWN TROUT
(*Salmo trutta*)

The brown trout is actually a European immigrant, transplanted to the United States late in the last century. Its present range includes the Northeast and down through the Appalachians, the upper Midwest, and mountainous regions of the West. The hardiest of all trout species, browns can withstand comparatively impure and warm water: 56 to 65 degrees F is their optimal temperature, but they can survive waters that heat up to the low 80s. In fact, brown trout have taken over many rivers and lakes in the eastern United States that, because of pollution, tree cutting, and other human impacts, can no longer support our native brook trout.

Brown trout can be difficult to catch and thus can grow to spectacular sizes, especially in large waters such as some Great Lakes. Average size depends on the habitat: from one half to two pounds in rivers, double that in still waters. Larger specimens are very often taken in both water types. The record brown trout was caught in 1992 in Little Red River, Arkansas, and weighed forty pounds four ounces.

For all the difficulty in getting them to hit your bait or lure, brown trout eat a wide variety of organisms: aquatic and terrestrial insects, crustaceans, small fish (even their own young), frogs,

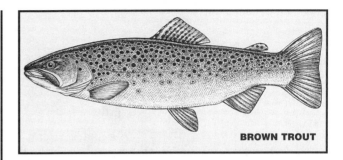

BROWN TROUT

and mice. The challenge in catching brown trout is twofold: they are highly nocturnal creatures, and they can be very selective when a particular food source presents itself in abundance, such as mayflies or stoneflies during a hatch.

The best lure and bait choices for brown trout depend entirely on the habitat and the time of year. Generally, live bait, such as garden worms and small minnows, and artificials, such as spinners and small spoons, work well, especially early and late in the year in rivers and smaller lakes. Fly fishermen do well with nymphs and streamers in early spring and move to wet and dry flies when insect hatches occur. In large lakes and reservoirs, fishing live bait—especially the prominent forage type, such as smelt—will take browns, as will trolling crankbaits and spoons imitating the forage.

RAINBOW TROUT
(*Oncorhynchus mykiss*)

If you hook a trout and it jumps out of the water frequently and spectacularly, chances are good it's a rainbow. This trout species is native to the Pacific drainage of the United States, but transplanting has increased the rainbow's range throughout the West and parts of the East and Midwest. Some rainbow trout are migratory—spending part of their lives in the ocean or one of the Great Lakes, and ascending freshwater streams to spawn—and these are called steelhead.

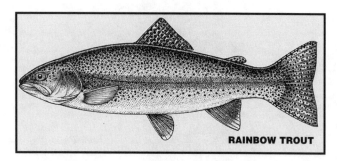

RAINBOW TROUT

Rainbow trout require clean, cold, well-oxygenated water and, in rivers, show a preference for fast-moving riffles and runs. Rainbows in lakes have similar needs and they will ascend tributaries if present to spawn. You will find rainbows in waters with temperatures ranging from 50 to 70 degrees F and a bit higher, but these fish favor temperatures in the upper 50s.

Rainbows average from half a pound to a couple of pounds in rivers and about twice that in lakes. Steelhead run much larger. The largest rainbow on record is a steelhead, caught in 1993 in Lake Michigan. It weighed thirty-one pounds six ounces.

Rainbow trout are usually not as difficult to catch as are brown trout, but they certainly aren't pushovers. The majority of a rainbow trout's diet is aquatic insects (which, along with their acrobatics, makes them a favorite of fly fishermen), but they will readily feed on terrestrial insects, worms, and small fish. Fly rodders should try to "match the hatch" if one is present; if not, brightly colored wet flies or streamers are a good bet. Spin fishermen do well with the baits mentioned above, as well as with brightly colored spinners and small spoons. Rainbows and steelhead also display a liking for fish roe, so baits such as salmon eggs and egg sacs are worth trying. In large lakes, rainbows and steelhead are usually caught by anglers fishing with live bait and/or lures that resemble the particular forage base in that water, such as alewives.

LAKE TROUT
(*Salvelinus namaycush*)

Actually a member of the char family, the lake trout is a denizen of deep, clear, cold lakes of the northern states and of some of the Great Lakes, and has been introduced into some waters of the western states. Generally bottom-oriented fish, lake trout can be caught in twenty feet of water early in the year, but later move to the depths—up to one hundred feet, with some subspecies moving as deep as five hundred feet. Temperatures at these depths are predictably cold; lake trout tend to inhabit waters in the 40- to 55-degree range and show a preference for waters from 48 to 52 degrees.

Because of the short "growing season" in their region, lake trout don't get big very quickly. However, they do reach impressive sizes. Average size depends largely on the locale—from two to five pounds or so is typical—but the world record lake trout, caught in Great Bear Lake, Northwest Territories, Canada, in 1991, weighed sixty-six pounds eight ounces. Commercial fishermen have caught lake trout weighing more than one hundred pounds.

Lake trout can be caught by fly fishermen and light-spin-tackle anglers in spring when the fish move to shallow water. Best offerings to use at this time are minnow simulations: streamers, spinners, spoons, and diving crankbaits. But the

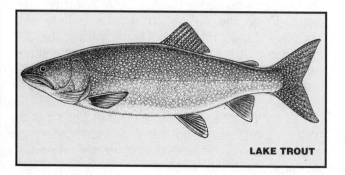

LAKE TROUT

majority of lake-trout fishing is done at depth by trolling with large spoons and live bait, such as smelt. In the past, heavy, unwieldy conventional rods and reels outfitted with wire line were necessary to reach the depths required. However, the advent of downriggers has allowed comparatively light-tackle anglers to fish for lake trout successfully.

BROOK TROUT
(*Salvelinus fontinalis*)

Also a member of the char family (though not referred to as one), the brookie is native to the northeast, the Appalachian Mountains, and parts of the north central United States. A stunningly beautiful fish, the brook trout is also the most demanding—perhaps "delicate" is a better term—regarding water quality. These fish need nearly pure water with a temperature that does not stray

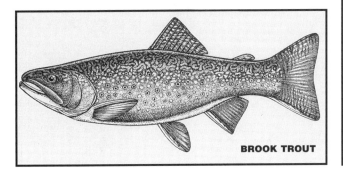

BROOK TROUT

too far from their preferred 45- to 61-degree F range, with 52 to 56 degrees being optimal. Although its name suggests a running water habitat (and most brookies these days are found in small, usually mountainous streams), brookies dwell in ponds and lakes that have an incoming source of cold water, such as a tributary or a spring. Unfortunately, the encroachment of civilization has severely cut back the brook trout's range, though stocking efforts by state fisheries departments allow a put-and-take brook trout fishery in many areas.

Native brook trout in streams may average only six inches or so (but these streams may be only six feet wide). In lakes, brook trout grow to larger sizes, though still not as big as other trout species. The largest brook trout on record was caught back in 1916 in the Nipigon River in Ontario, Canada, and weighed fourteen pounds eight ounces. It is doubtful that this record will ever be beaten.

Brookies eat a variety of forage, though in most places it is limited to aquatic and terrestrial insects, baitfish, and crustaceans. Brookies are not considered difficult to catch, though at times these fish will "turn off" and frustrate even the most dedicated fishermen. In streams, fly fishermen should use bright wet flies, small streamers, and nymphs; spin fishermen do well with live bait such as garden worms and small minnows, as well as miniature spinners and spoons. Baits and lures for lakes are similar and can be somewhat larger.

APPENDIX 1
BOAT MANUFACTURERS

Note: This is not comprehensive, as no master list of every manufacturer of freshwater fishing boats exists, but the author has striven to make it as complete as possible.

Achilles Inflatable Craft
1407 80th St. SW
Everett, WA 98203
206/353-7000
Inflatable boats

Actioncraft Inc.
2603 Andalusia Blvd.
Cape Coral, FL 33909
813/574-7008
Fiberglass flats/bass boats

Allison Boats, Inc.
106 Main St.
Louisville, TN 37777
615/983-5920
Fiberglass bass boats

Alumacraft Boat Co.
315 W. St. Juline St.
St. Peter, MN 56082
507/931-1050
Aluminum bass boats, multispecies boats

Aquasport Marine (Genmar)
1651 Whitfield Ave.
Sarasota, FL 34243
813/755-5800
Fiberglass console boats

Astro Boats (Brunswick Marine)
6776 Old Nashville Hwy.
Murfreesboro, TN 37130
615/890-1593
Fiberglass bass boats, multispecies boats, fish/ski sport boats

Bass Cat Boats
P.O. Drawer 1360
Mountain Home, AR 72653
501/481-5135
Bass boats

Bayliner Marine Corp. (Brunswick Marine)
P.O. Box 9029
Everett, WA 98206
206/435-6534
Fiberglass fish/ski sport boats

Boston Whaler, Inc.
4121 South U.S. Hwy. 1
Edgewater, FL 32141
904/426-1400
Fiberglass utility boats, flats boats

Bullet Boats Inc.
P.O. Box 2202
Knoxville, TN 37901
615/577-7055
Fiberglass bass boats

Cajun Boats (Genmar)
3200 Industrial Dr.
Winnsboro, LA 71295
318/435-9431
Fiberglass bass boats, multispecies boats, console boats

Carolina Skiff
3231 Fulford Rd.
Waycross, GA 31503
912/287-0547
Fiberglass utility boats, console boats

Celebrity Boats, Inc.
P.O. Box 394
451 E. Illinois Ave.
Benton, IL 62812
618/439-9444
Fiberglass console boats

Century Boat Co.
6725 Bay Line Dr.
Panama City, FL 32406
904/769-0311
Fiberglass console boats

Champion Boats, Inc.
P.O. Box 3900
Mountain Home, AR 72653
501/425-8188
Fiberglass bass boats, multispecies boats,
fish/ski sport boats

Charger Boats/Play Craft Boats/RichLine Boats
P.O. Box 709
Richland, MO 65556
314/765-3265
Fiberglass and aluminum bass boats, pontoon
boats

Cobia Boat Co. (Caribbean Boats)
2000 Cobia Dr.
Vonore, TN 37885
615/884-6881
Fiberglass console boats

Crestliner Boats (Genmar)
609 13th Ave. N.E.
Little Falls, MN 56345
1-800/889-7020
Aluminum console boats, pontoon boats

Discovery Marine Inc.
2090 Preble Rd.
Preble, NY 13141
607/749-7960
Aluminum utility boats, multispecies boats,
console boats, pontoon boats

Duracraft Boats
125 Superior Dr.
Delhi, LA 71232
318/878-2628
Aluminum utility boats, console boats

Fisher Boats (Brunswick Marine)
P.O. Box 517
Topeka, IN 46571
1-800/622-8181
Aluminum utility bass boats, johnboats,
multispecies boats, pontoon boats

Four Winns (OMC FBG)
925 Frisbie
Cadillac, MI 49601
616/775-1351
Fiberglass fish/ski sport boats

Grady-White Boats
P.O. Box 1527
Grenville, NC 27835
919/752-2111
Fiberglass console boats

Grumman Boats (OMC ABG)
2900 Industrial Dr.
Lebanon, MO 65536
1-800/662-4386
Aluminum utility boats, johnboats, bass boats,
multispecies boats, pontoon boats

Grumman Canoes (OMC ABG)
P.O. Box 549
Marathon, NY 13803
607/849-3211
Aluminum canoes

Hydra-Sports (OMC FBG)
880 Butler Rd.
Murfreesboro, TN 37130
615/895-5190
Fiberglass bass boats, fish/ski sport boats,
console boats, flats boats

Javelin Boats (OMC FBG)
880 Butler Rd.
Murfreesboro, TN 37130
615/895-5190
Fiberglass bass boats, multispecies boats

Kenner Manufacturing Co.
No. 2 Red Barn Rd.
Knoxville, AR 72845
501/885-3171
Fiberglass console boats

Lowe Aluminum Boats (OMC ABG)
2900 Industrial Dr.
Lebanon, MO 65536
1-800/662-4386
Aluminum utility boats, johnboats, bass boats, multispecies boats, pontoon boats

Luhrs Corp.
255 Diesel Rd.
St. Augustine, FL 32086
1-800/829-5847
Fiberglass console boats

Lund Boat Division (Genmar)
P.O. Box 248
New York Mills, MN 56567
218/385-2235
Aluminum utility boats, multispecies boats, console boats, pontoon boats

Mako Marine
4355 N.W. 128th St.
Miami, FL 33054
305/685-6591
Fiberglass console boats, flats boats

Maritec Industries, Inc. (Gambler Bass Boats)
5980 Lakehurst Dr.
Orlando, FL 32809
407/352-6066
Fiberglass bass boats

Maritime International, Inc.
P.O. Box 218
Duxbury, MA 02331
617/934-0010
Fiberglass console boats

MonArk Boats (Brunswick Marine)
P.O. Box 517
Topeka, IN 46571
1-800/622-8181
Aluminum utility bass boats, johnboats, multi-species boats, pontoon boats

Nitro High Performance Boats (Tracker Marine)
Bass Pro Shops
1935 S. Campbell
Springfield, MO 65898
417/882-4000
Fiberglass bass boats

Polar Kraft Mfg. Co.
9570 Lamar Ave.
Olive Branch, MS 38654
601/895-5576
Bass America boats: aluminum bass boats, multispecies boats, utility boats

Porta-Bote International
1074 Independence Ave.
Mountain View, CA 94043
415/961-5334
Folding utility boats

Premier Pontoon Boats
26430 Fallbrook Ave.
Wyoming, MN 55092
612/462-2880
Pontoon boats

Princecraft U.S. (OMC)
200 Sea Horse Dr.
Waukegan, IL 60085
708/689-5580
Aluminum utility boats, console boats, bass boats, multispecies boats

ProCraft Boats (Brunswick Marine)
6776 Old Nashville Hwy.
Murfreesboro, TN 37130
615/890-1593
Fiberglass bass boats, multispecies boats, fish/ski sport boats

Pro-Line Boats, Inc.
Box 1348
Crystal River, FL 34423
1-800/866-2771
Fiberglass console boats, flats boats

Pursuit Fishing Boats
3901 St. Lucie Blvd.
Fort Pierce, FL 34946
407/465-6006
Fiberglass console boats

Quest Boats (OMC FBG)
880 Butler Rd.
Murfreesboro, TN 37130
615/895-5190
Fiberglass console boats

Quicksilver (Brunswick Marine)
P.O. Box 1939
Fond du Lac, WI 54936
414/929-5000
Inflatable boats

Ranger Boats (Genmar)
P.O. Box 179
Flippin, AR 72634
501/453-2222
Fiberglass bass boats, multispecies boats,
fish/ski sport boats, flats boats, console boats

Roughneck Aluminum Boats (OMC ABG)
2900 Industrial Dr.
Lebanon, MO 65536
1-800/662-4386
Aluminum johnboats, bass boats

SeaArk Boats, Inc.
P.O. Box 803
Monticello, AR 71655
501/367-5317
Aluminum johnboats, bass boats, console
boats

Sea Nymph Boats (OMC ABG)
2900 Industrial Dr.
Lebanon, MO 65536
1-800/662-4386
Aluminum utility boats, johnboats, console
boats, bass boats, multispecies boats, pontoon boats

Sea Ray Boats Inc. (Brunswick Marine)
2600 Sea Ray Blvd.
Knoxville, TN 37914
1-800/772-6287
Laguna boats: fiberglass console boats

Sears, Roebuck and Co.
1630 Cleveland Ave.
Kansas City, MO 64127
1-800/366-3000
Gamefisher aluminum utility boats, johnboats,
fiberglass canoes

Seaswirl Boats (OMC)
P.O. Box 167
Culver, OR 97734
503/546-5011
Fiberglass console boats

Skeeter Products Inc.
P.O. Box 230
Kilgore, TX 75663
903/984-0541
Fiberglass bass boats, fish/ski sport boats

Smoker Craft/Sylvan Marine
P.O. Box 65
New Paris, IN 46553
219/831-2103
Aluminum utility boats, bass boats, johnboats,
multispecies boats, pontoon boats

Spectrum Boats (Brunswick Marine)
P.O. Box 517
Topeka, IN 46571
1-800/622-8181
Aluminum utility boats, bass boats, johnboats,
multispecies boats, pontoon boats

Starcraft (Brunswick Marine)
201 Starcraft Dr.
Topeka, IN 46571
1-800/622-8181
Aluminum utility boats, bass boats, multispecies boats, console boats, pontoon boats

Stratos Boats (OMC FBG)
931 Industrial Rd.
Old Hickory, TN 37138
615/847-4034
Fiberglass console boats, bass boats, fish/ski sport boats, multispecies boats

Sunbird Boat Co., Inc. (OMC)
2348 Shop Rd.
Columbia, SC 29201
803/799-1125
Fiberglass console boats, pontoon boats

Suncruiser Pontoons (OMC ABG)
2900 Industrial Dr.
Lebanon, MO 65536
1-800/662-4386
Aluminum pontoon boats

Sun Tracker Pontoon Boats (Tracker Marine)
Bass Pro Shops
1935 S. Campbell
Springfield, MO 65898
417/882-4000
Aluminum pontoon boats

Tracker Boats (Tracker Marine)
Bass Pro Shops
1935 S. Campbell
Springfield, MO 65898
417/882-4000
Aluminum bass boats, multispecies boats

Tri-State Custom Fiberglass Co. (Hawk Boats)
P.O. Box 369
Bailey, NC 27807
919/235-2461
Fiberglass console boats

Wahoo Boats Unlimited
708 Air Park Rd.
Ashland, VA 23005
804/798-2780
Fiberglass console boats

Water Moccasin Boats Inc.
Rte. 1, Box 957
Stonewall, LA 71078
318/925-9668
Fiberglass "personal watercraft"

Wellcraft Boats (Genmar)
1651 Whitfield Ave.
Sarasota, FL 34243
1-800/923-9000
Fiberglass console boats

Yar-Craft Inc.
1213 20th Ave.
Menominee, MI 49858
906/863-4497
Fiberglass console boats, multispecies boats

Zodiac of North America
Thompson Creek Rd.
Stevensville, MD 21666
410/643-4141
Inflatable boats

Guide

Brunswick Marine: A division of the Brunswick Corporation.
OMC: A division of Outboard Marine Corporation, Inc.
OMC ABG: A division of Outboard Marine Corporation Aluminum Boat Group, Inc.
OMC FBG: A division of Outboard Marine Corporation Fishing Boat Group, Inc.
Genmar: A division of Genmar Industries, Inc.

APPENDIX 2
OUTBOARD MOTOR MANUFACTURERS

American Honda Marine Corp.
4475 River Green Pkwy.
Duluth, GA 30136
404/497-6066
Honda outboards

American Suzuki Motor Corp.
3251 East Imperial Hwy.
Brea, CA 92621
1-800/447-2882
Suzuki outboards

Mercury Marine (Brunswick Marine)
W6250 W. Pioneer Rd.
P.O. Box 1939
Fond du Lac, WI 54936
414/929-5060
Mercury/Mariner/Force outboards

Outboard Marine Corp. (OMC)
Marine Power Products Group
200 Sea Horse Dr.
Waukegan, IL 60085
1-800/998-9960
Evinrude outboards, Johnson outboards

Sears, Roebuck and Co.
1630 Cleveland Ave.
Kansas City, MO 64127
1-800/366-3000
Gamefisher outboard motors

Tohatsu Corporation
Tohatsu East
500 Marathon Pkwy., NW
Arbor Business Park
Lawrenceville, GA 30245
404/339-3510

Tohatsu West
984 N. Lemon
Orange, CA 92667
714/744-1084
Tohatsu outboards

Yamaha Motor Corp. USA
Marine Group
P.O. Box 6555
Cypress, GA 90630
1-800/526-6650
Yamaha outboards

Yanmar Diesel America Corp.
901 Corporate Grove Dr.
Buffalo Grove, IL 60069
708/541-1900
Yanmar diesel outboards

INDEX

Picture Credits

Bayliner Marine, 8, 18; Brunswick Marine, 10; Crestliner Boats, 4 (lower right); Furino, 54; Honda Marine, 35 (upper left); Humminbird, 55; Marine Power Inc., 35 (right); OMC Fishing Boat Group, 5 (both); Outboard Marine Corporation, 30; Piranha Propellers, 37 (bottom); Porta-Bote International, 25 (both); Propco Marine Propellers, 37 (top); Ranger Boats, 12; Sunbird Boat Company, 17; Tohatsu Outboards, 29, 31; Zodiak of North America, 23. The remaining photographs are by the author of this book.

The following people participated in the preparation of this book: Michael Burke, Martin Dowding, Mimi Maxwell, Eileen Morin, Tom Nau, and Alison Reid.